MW00745262

Inside—Find the Answers to These Questions and More

☑ Is osteoporosis becoming an epidemic? (See page 12.)

☑ Who is at the greatest risk for osteoporosis? (See page 15.)

☑ What is osteoporosis, and how does it develop? (See page 1.)

☑ What are the benefits and risks of estrogen replacement therapy for preventing osteoporosis? (See page 132.)

☑ Is ipriflavone—a substance derived from compounds in soybeans—a safe and effective alternative to estrogen? (See page 73.)

☑ How do calcium and vitamin D fight osteoporosis? (See page 42.)

☑ Which other nutrients are important for your bones' health? (See page 86.)

☑ Is fast food dangerous for your bones? (See page 109.)

☑ What is the best way to determine your personal risk for osteoporosis? (See page 143.)

☑ How can you protect and even rebuild weakened bone *before* you try a medication or nutritional supplement? (See page 104.)

THE NATURAL PHARMACIST™ Library

Natural Health Bible
Your Complete Guide to Illnesses and
Their Natural Remedies
Your Complete Guide to Herbs
Your Complete Guide to Vitamins and Supplements
Feverfew and Migraines
Heart Disease Prevention
Kava and Anxiety
Arthritis
Colds and Flus
Diabetes
Osteoporosis
Garlic and Cholesterol
Ginkgo and Memory
Menopause
PMS
Reducing Cancer Risk
Saw Palmetto and the Prostate
St. John's Wort and Depression
Preventing Osteoporosis with Ipriflavone

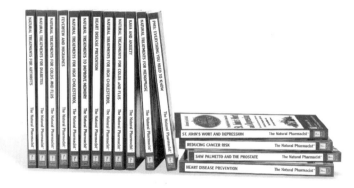

Visit us online at www.TNP.com

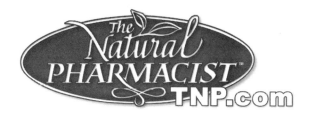

Everything You Need to Know About

Osteoporosis

Sheila Dunn-Merritt, N.D.
& Lyn Patrick, N.D.

Edited by

Carol Poole

Andrea Girman, M.D., M.P.H

Series Editors

Steven Bratman, M.D.

David Kroll, Ph.D.

A DIVISION OF PRIMA PUBLISHING

3000 Lava Ridge Court ■ Roseville, California 95661

(800) 632-8676 ■ www.primahealth.com

Published in association with TNP.com.

Warning—Disclaimer
This book is not intended to provide medical advice and is sold with the understanding that the publisher and the author are not liable for the misconception or misuse of information provided. The author and Prima Publishing shall have neither liability nor responsibility to any person or entity with respect to any loss, damage, or injury caused or alleged to be caused directly or indirectly by the information contained in this book or the use of any products mentioned. Readers should not use any of the products discussed in this book without the advice of a medical professional.

TNP.COM, THENATURALPHARMACIST.COM, THE NATURAL PHARMACIST, and associated logos are trademarks of Prima Communications Inc. The Prima Health logo is a registered trademark of Prima Communications Inc., registered with the United States Patent and Trademark Office.

The Food and Drug Administration has not approved the use of any of the natural treatments discussed in this book. This book, and the information contained herein, has not been approved by the Food and Drug Administration.

Pseudonyms have been used throughout to protect the privacy of the individuals involved.

All products mentioned in this book are trademarks of their respective companies.

Illustrations © 2000 by Prima Publishing. All rights reserved.

Library of Congress Cataloging-in-Publication Data on File
CIP 00-105937
ISBN 0-7615-1618-2

00 01 02 03 HH 10 9 8 7 6 5 4 3 2 1
Printed in the United States of America

How to Order
Single copies may be ordered from Prima Publishing, 3000 Lava Ridge Court, Roseville, CA 95661; telephone (800) 632-8676 ext. 4444. Quantity discounts are also available. On your letterhead, include information concerning the intended use of the books and the number of books you wish to purchase.

**Visit us online at www.TNP.com and
www.primahealth.com**

Contents

What Makes This Book Different?

The interest in natural medicine has never been greater. According to the National Association of Chain Drug Stores, 65 million Americans are using natural supplements, and the number is growing! Yet, it is hard for the consumer to find trustworthy sources for balanced information about this emerging field. Why? Frankly, natural medicine has had a checkered history. From snake oil potions sold at the turn of the century to those books, magazines, and product catalogs that hype miracle cures today, this is a field where exaggerated claims have been the norm. Proponents of natural medicine have tended to abuse science, treating it more as a marketing tool than a means of discovering the truth.

But there is truth to be found. Studies of vitamins, minerals, and other food supplements have been with us since these nutritional substances were first discovered, and the level and quality of this science has grown dramatically in the last 20 years. Herbal medicine has been neglected in the United States, but in Europe, this, the oldest of all healing arts, has been the subject of tremendous and ongoing scientific interest.

At present, for a number of herbs and supplements, it is possible to give reasonably scientific answers to the questions: How well does this work? How safe is it? What types of conditions is it best used for?

THE NATURAL PHARMACIST series is designed to cut through the hype and tell you what is known and what remains to be scientifically proven regarding popular natural treatments. These books are more conservative than any others available, more honest about the weaknesses of natural approaches, more fair in their comparisons of natural and conventional treatments. You won't find any miracle cures here, but you will discover useful options that can help you become healthier.

Why Choose Natural Treatments?

Although the science behind natural medicine continues to grow, this is still a much less scientifically validated field than conventional medicine. You might ask, "Why should I resort to an herb that is only partly proven, when I could take a drug with solid science behind it?" There are at least three good reasons to consider natural alternatives.

First, some herbs and supplements offer benefits that are not matched by any conventional drug. Vitamin E is a good example. It appears to help prevent prostate cancer, a benefit that no standard medication can claim.

Another example is the herb milk thistle. Studies strongly suggest that this herb can protect the liver from injury. There is no pill or tablet your doctor can prescribe to do the same.

Even if the science behind some of these treatments is less than perfect, when the risks are low and the possible benefit high, a natural treatment may be worth trying. It is a little-known fact that for many conventional treatments the science is less than perfect as well, and physicians must balance uncertain benefits against incompletely understood risks.

A second reason to consider natural therapies is that some may offer benefits comparable to those of drugs with fewer side effects. The herb St. John's wort is a good example. Reasonably strong scientific evidence suggests that this herb is an effective treatment for mild to moderate depression, while producing fewer side effects on average than conventional medications. Saw palmetto for benign enlargement of the prostate, ginkgo for relieving symptoms and perhaps slowing the progression of Alzheimer's disease, and glucosamine for osteoarthritis are other examples. This is not to say that herbs and supplements are completely harmless—they're not—but for most the level of risk is quite low.

Finally, there is a philosophical point to consider. For many people, it "feels" better to use a treatment that comes from nature instead of from a laboratory. Just as you might rather wear all-cotton clothing than polyester, or look at a mountain landscape rather than the skyscrapers of a downtown city, natural treatments may simply feel more compatible with your view of life. We can quibble endlessly about just what "natural" means and whether a certain treatment is "actually" natural or not, but such arguments are beside the point. The difference is in the feeling, and feelings matter. In fact, having a good feeling about taking an herb may lead you to use it more consistently than you would a prescription drug.

Of course, at times synthetic drugs may be necessary and even lifesaving. But on many other occasions it may be quite reasonable to turn to an herb or supplement instead of a drug.

To make good decisions you need good information. Unfortunately, while hundreds of books on alternative medicine are published every year, many are highly misleading. The phrase "studies prove" is often used when the studies in question are so small or so badly conducted that they prove nothing at all. You may even find that the "data" from other books comes from studies with petri dishes and not real people!

You can't even assume that books written by well-known authors are scientifically sound. Many of these authors rely on secondary writers, leading to a game of "telephone," where misconceptions are passed around from book to book. And there's a strong tendency to exaggerate the power of natural remedies, whitewashing them with selective reporting.

THE NATURAL PHARMACIST series gives you the balanced information you need to make informed decisions about your health needs. Setting a new, high standard of accuracy and objectivity, these books take a realistic look at the herbs and supplements you read about in the news. You will encounter both favorable and unfavorable studies in these pages and will learn about both the benefits and the risks of natural treatments.

THE NATURAL PHARMACIST series is the source you can trust.

Steven Bratman, M.D.
David Kroll, Ph.D.

Introduction

Osteoporosis is a serious disease that causes the bones to become progressively lighter and weaker until they are dangerously easy to break, especially in the hips, spine, and wrists. Men and women of all ages and races get osteoporosis, but some groups have a higher risk than others.

Modern medicine is helping people live longer and healthier lives, yet the fact that we can expect to live longer also means that we're at greater risk for eventually suffering from osteoporosis. Osteoporosis is becoming even more widespread as baby boomers approach menopause and their senior years, and the elderly population is projected to grow for decades to come. According to current estimates, nearly 1 in 4 women over age 65 will have osteoporosis. For women over 80, this figure rises to 1 in 2. Although the vast majority of people with osteoporosis are women, 1 in 10 men over age 80 get this disease, too. Today, 28 million Americans are at high risk for osteoporosis. Every year, an estimated 250,000 Americans suffer a broken hip; about 50% of the time, a broken hip leads to a permanent loss of independence and ability. The complications from these fractures (infections, pneumonia, blood clots, etc.) are the reason that falls are the number one cause of accidental death in people over 75.

By the year 2001, these fractures will cost our health care system $30 to $40 billion each year.

Modern diagnostic tools have made it possible to detect and treat osteoporosis long before it causes a broken bone. As yet, there is no single cure for osteoporosis. This disease is caused by many factors, including the normal processes of aging and the hormonal changes that naturally occur with menopause.

A number of medications can protect against bone loss, and some can even rebuild bones to make them stronger. But because osteoporosis is a complex disease, influenced by diet, nutrition, lifestyle, certain medications, and other known factors, it makes sense to use a holistic, preventive approach. The following sections describe a number of natural alternatives, including dietary supplements and changes you can make in your lifestyle, that have been proven effective in protecting against bone loss and reducing your risk for osteoporosis.

What Is Osteoporosis?

O steoporosis is a serious disease that affects 20% of women and 5% of men aged 50 and over in the United States.[1] Literally meaning "porous bone," osteoporosis is a condition in which your bones actually lose mass and density while their structure changes, becoming progressively weaker and more brittle until they're dangerously prone to break.

Men and women of all ages can get osteoporosis.[2] (See chapter 2, Who Is at Risk?) Poor nutrition and certain diseases can cause osteoporosis at any age. But in general, osteoporosis is most common among older people, especially postmenopausal women. Not long ago, it was considered normal for an older woman to lose inches of height or acquire a "dowager's hump" as the bones of her spine fractured from osteoporosis. (We're glad to say that this is no longer considered a normal part of aging, thanks to the therapies you'll read about in the following chapters.)

Although more women than men get osteoporosis, it's important to realize that the impact on men is significant,

The Silent Disease

A 92-year-old woman, Helen, went to her doctor complaining of back pain. Though she'd had a mild stroke three years earlier and needed a walker or a wheelchair, she'd remained active and cheerful. But now her back was so sore, she said, that she couldn't find a comfortable position to sit in. Weeks of physical therapy, massage, ice packs, and anti-inflammatory medications hadn't helped. Helen was at her wits' end.

At her doctor's suggestion, x rays were taken. They revealed that Helen had a collapsed bone in her spine, commonly called a "compression fracture."

When the bones of the spinal column are weakened by osteoporosis, a simple action like bending forward to make a bed or lifting a heavy pan out of the oven can actually result in such a fracture, causing back pain, decreased height, or the curved spine known as a "dowager's hump."

Unfortunately, many women don't realize they have osteoporosis until a simple everyday action breaks a bone in their wrist or spine. This is why it's called "the silent disease."

too, especially after age 70. In fact, American men over age 50 are more likely to suffer an osteoporosis-related fracture than to develop clinical prostate cancer, according to the National Osteoporosis Foundation (www.nof.org).[3]

How Is Bone Made?

Of course, you know that your bones are the strong, hard structures that protect certain organs and give your body its fundamental shape. But you may not know that your bones are continually going through a process called *remodeling,* in which old bone cells are destroyed and new ones created. Although we may think of it as a fixed, inanimate thing, bone is actually living tissue that is continually changing. Like muscle, it gets larger and stronger when you use it more strenuously, and weaker when it's not used. (For more information, see chapter 7, Exercise, Diet, and Lifestyle: What You Can Do to Protect Your Bones.)

Although we may think of it as a fixed, inanimate thing, bone is actually living tissue that is continually changing.

Bone is made of tiny crystals of *calcium* and *phosphorus,* as well as *collagen* and other proteins and minerals. Calcium is a mineral that most people are familiar with; it gives bone its hard, dense solidness. Collagen, a protein also found in skin and scar tissue, surrounds the crystals and gives bone a certain amount of flexibility and suppleness. You may not think of your bones as being very flexible, but much of their strength actually comes from the collagen that lets them absorb considerable shock before they break. Your bones also contain other minerals such as calcium phosphate, calcium carbonate, and small amounts of magnesium, fluoride, sulfate, and other trace minerals.

There are two kinds of bone tissue. Compact (or *cortical*) bone makes up the major part of the long bones of the arms and legs and the outermost layer of most bones. As its name suggests, compact bone is hard and dense. About 80% of your bone tissue is compact bone.[4] The other type of bone tissue is known as spongy (or *trabecular*) bone. Spongy bone is a fine lattice network that surrounds the bone *marrow,* the soft fatty tissue that

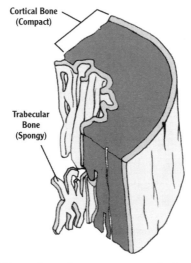

Figure 1.   *The cross section of a bone*

produces blood cells.[4] In the long bones of the arms and legs, spongy bone appears mainly at the ends (the wrists and hips). But the vertebrae in your spine are mostly composed of spongy bone. Its structure provides maximum support with minimal bone material (see figure 1).

Both types of bone tissue are constantly being broken down and replaced by natural processes in the body. This cycle of bone remodeling helps us in several ways. It allows our bodies to build up the strength of bones we use in intense activity. It also protects us against the cumulative effects of stress.

Imagine an old china plate, lined with tiny hairline fractures from years of use. If you dropped the plate on the floor it would certainly shatter. Unlike this plate, your bones are constantly renewing themselves, replacing stressed bone tissue with fresh new cells and healing any microscopic fractures that might develop. This is perhaps the

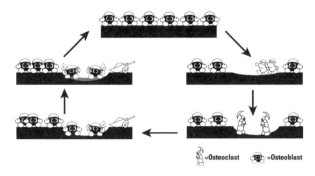

Figure 2. *The bone remodeling cycle*

most important benefit we get from the continual process of bone remodeling—it keeps bones new and strong.

Bone remodeling has two phases: tearing down, and building up. In the first phase, the parathyroid gland signals the body to release a type of cell called *osteoclasts.* These cells selectively break down, or *resorb,* bone cells. Then in the second phase, the thyroid gland secretes a hormone called calcitonin, signaling the release of cells called *osteoblasts.* These osteoblasts build new bone cells to replace the old (see figure 2).

To build new bone, your body needs a good supply of calcium and other essential minerals. To learn more about the role of nutrition in maintaining bone health, see the chapters Calcium and Vitamin D for Osteoporosis, Other Important Nutrients for Your Bones, and Exercise, Diet, and Lifestyle: What You Can Do to Protect Your Bones.

Your Bones Are a Storehouse

Of course, your bones give your body strength and structure, but you may not know that they play another important role, which is serving as a storehouse of essential minerals. Your bones are made of calcium plus collagen and other proteins and minerals. In fact, more than 99% of the calcium in your body is contained in your bones and teeth. But the remaining tiny fraction of calcium is extremely important. Every system and process in your body needs calcium. Without it, your muscles couldn't contract, your blood wouldn't clot, and your heart wouldn't beat.

What happens when your blood level of calcium falls too low to meet your body's needs? This can happen if you aren't getting enough calcium in your diet, if something is interfering with your ability to absorb it from your food, or if you are losing a lot of calcium in your urine (this can happen if you eat a high-salt diet). The answer is that, when it has to, your body can get calcium from your bones. When your blood level of calcium falls below a certain level, a complex mechanism in your body restores your level of calcium. If necessary, it sacrifices some of your bone tissue to release calcium back into your blood.

While this mechanism is good to have in an emergency, you obviously don't want to encourage your body to break down bone tissue for any reason. It's much better to make sure your diet is giving you all the calcium you need in the first place. The chapters Calcium and Vitamin D for Osteoporosis and Other Important Nutrients for Your Bones discuss in greater detail how calcium, vitamin D, and other vitamins and minerals can help protect you against osteoporosis.

What Is the Life Cycle of Bone?

In the earliest years of our lives, our bodies build more new bone than they resorb. New bone is built on the outer surface of the bones and resorbed from the inner surface. We continue to build more bone than we lose until around age 20 to 25, which is when our bones achieve their highest level of size and density—our *peak bone mass*.

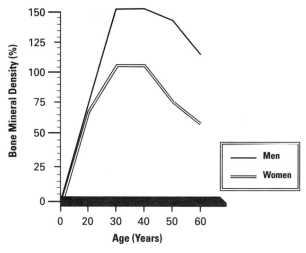

Figure 3. *Bone mineral density in men and women*

In general, the greater your peak bone mass, the more bone you can afford to lose before you develop osteoporosis. Since peak bone mass is built so early in life, it's important that children and teens get the nutrition and exercise their bones need. For more information about peak bone mass, see the chapters Who Is at Risk? and Other Important Nutrients for Your Bones.

What happens after you've achieved your peak bone mass in your early 20s? For several years, nothing much changes. Your body makes just about enough new bone to replace the old. The density and mass of your bones remains stable or declines slightly. Men and women in their 40s begin to lose about 0.3% to 0.5% of their bone mass each year (see figure 3).[5]

It's too bad that the life cycle of bone doesn't end here, but there's a third stage. After menopause, the rate of bone loss in women increases dramatically for several years. For men, too, bone loss speeds up at about age 50, although not as dramatically. In either case, the result is that we *lose* as much as 1% to 2% of total bone mass each year.

This natural process doesn't necessarily lead all the way to osteoporosis. If you start out with a high peak bone mass, a gradual yearly bone loss may never add up to dangerous levels. However, if you lose 1% of your bone mass each year for 20 or 30 years, the cumulative loss can be severe, especially if your peak bone mass was less than optimal. Chapter 2, Who Is at Risk?, explains why some people may be at higher risk than others for osteoporosis.

Throughout its life cycle, bone is shaped, built up, and torn down by hormones. The body uses calcitonin and other hormones to start and finish the bone remodeling process. For women, the sex hormone *estrogen* plays a major role in generally protecting bone mass. This means that a woman's bones may be greatly affected by the hormonal changes of menopause.

How Does Menopause Cause Bone Loss to Accelerate?

When a woman enters menopause, her body's production of estrogen slows dramatically. (In men, sex hormones decline with age, too, but more gradually.)

Estrogen is a hormone that plays many key roles in the body. Among its numerous jobs, one of its lesser-known duties is to maintain the body's normal rate of bone remodeling. When the level of estrogen drops after menopause, a woman's body begins to resorb bone much faster than she rebuilds it.

Unless a woman takes supplemental hormones or uses an appropriate natural therapy, the result is an accelerated loss of bone—for some women, as much as 3 to 5% of bone mass or more *each year!*

This faster rate of bone loss continues for 3 to 6 years after menopause. Then, at around age 60 or 65, a woman's rate of bone loss slows to around the same rate as a man's of the same age: 1 to 2% each year on average.[6]

Is there some good reason why women's bones become weaker after menopause? We can only speculate about why our bodies do this. But we do know that estrogen is one of the key elements to this accelerated bone loss after menopause. Chapter 3, Menopause, Estrogen, and Osteoporosis, explains further the role that estrogen and other hormones play in protecting the size and density of your bones. Hormones and hormone-like substances are used in some of the leading conventional and alternative treatments to prevent osteoporosis. For information about these treatments, see the chapters Menopause, Estrogen, and Osteoporosis; Ipriflavone and Phytoestrogens; and Progesterone for Osteoporosis.

Unless a woman takes supplemental hormones or uses an appropriate natural therapy, the result is an accelerated loss of bone— for some women, as much as 3 to 5% of bone mass or more *each year!*

Wrists, Spine, and Hips: The Weak Links

Osteoporosis can occur anywhere in the body, but most fractures due to osteoporosis happen in the wrists, spine, and hips. To understand why, look again at the composition of bone (see figure 4). There are two types of bone tissue: compact (or *cortical*) and spongy (or *trabecular*).

Compact bone is particularly useful for its hardness and mass. The long bones of the arm and leg are made almost entirely of compact bone. Trabecular bone has a very

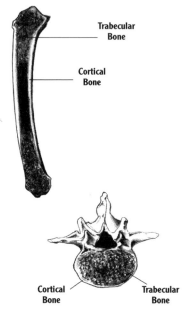

Figure 4.   *Cortical and trabecular tissue
in a tibia and a vertebra*

different, spongy structure that makes it ideal for with-
standing stress and providing flexible support. Unfortunately, it's also especially vulnerable to osteoporosis.

Only about 20% of your bone tissue is trabecular
bone, but it's concentrated in certain areas that are prone
to stress: the spine, and the ends of the long bones of the
arms and legs, at the wrists and hips. Your *vertebrae*
(bones of your spine) are made mostly of trabecular bone
covered by just a thin shell of compact (cortical) bone.

Due to the spongy texture of trabecular bone, it's
more vulnerable to osteoporosis. Spongy bone is made of
a relatively small amount of bone tissue spread out in a
lattice formation with lots of exposed surfaces. Compared
to compact bone, it has a higher rate of turnover in the

The Symptoms of Osteoporosis

Osteoporosis is often called "the silent disease" because in its early stages it has no symptoms. It can progress for decades before any noticeable symptoms appear. Once the disease is advanced, it may cause:

- Height loss
- Curving spine ("dowager's hump")
- Persistent back pain
- Muscle aches, pain, and spasms in the back
- Rib pain
- Tooth loss
- Fractures (especially the wrist, vertebra, and hip)

cycle of bone remodeling, and is more affected by the hormonal changes of menopause.[7]

Your spine, hips, and wrists are doubly vulnerable to fractures from osteoporosis, not only because of their higher concentration of spongy bone, but because they happen to be the areas where you are most likely to hurt yourself in everyday life. When you trip, you catch yourself with your hands, and your wrists absorb the impact. When you fall, you land on your hips. Whenever you sit, stand up, walk, or lie down, you make demands on your spine and hips. Osteoporosis robs your bones of the flexibility to withstand these everyday stresses and traumas.

It's not hard to see why osteoporosis turns everyday accidents into life-threatening disasters. According to the Osteoporosis and Related Bone Diseases-National Resource Center (www.osteo.org), in the United States alone osteoporosis is responsible for more than 1.5 million fractures each year, including 700,000 fractures of the vertebrae, 300,000 hip fractures, and 250,000 wrist fractures.[8]

For many people, a hip fracture can be a disabling catastrophe. Nearly 24% of elderly people who suffer one die within a year.[9] For many others, a fracture from osteoporosis leads to a permanent loss of independence and mobility. Most troubling of all, perhaps, is the startling statistic that Caucasian women in the United States have about the same risk of dying from an osteoporosis-related hip fractures as they do of dying from breast cancer.[10]

Is Osteoporosis an Epidemic?

The National Osteoporosis Foundation (www.nof.org) estimates that, of people over age 50, one of every two women and one in eight men will have an osteoporosis-related fracture in their lifetime.[11] Whether or not it's an "epidemic," osteoporosis is clearly a problem that has the potential to affect most families.

In his book *Preventing and Reversing Osteoporosis,* Dr. Alan R. Gaby argues that osteoporosis may be growing more common in the modern world. He describes a fascinating study that was reported in 1993 in the British medical journal *The Lancet.* In this study, skeletons dating from 1729 to 1852 were analyzed for the rate of bone loss in their hips. (The skeletons had been unearthed during the restoration of a church in London.) The rate of bone loss, before and after menopause, was much lower in the skeletons than for modern women in northern Europe.[12] Dr. Gaby also cites some studies from Sweden and England showing higher rates of osteoporosis-related fractures in 1980 or 1981 compared to earlier years (1971, 1956, and 1950).[13–15]

Does this mean that osteoporosis is becoming more common in the modern world? We don't know. It's certainly possible that some aspects of modern life may be increasing people's risk for osteoporosis. Your bones are strengthened and built up by intense exercise and weakened by a sedentary lifestyle (see chapter 7, Exercise, Diet, and Lifestyle: What You Can Do to Protect Your Bones). Most of us probably do less physical work than our grandparents did in their youth. It's also possible that certain types of environmental pollution, or features of the modern diet, might be harmful to bone. We *do* know that certain modern medications can cause osteoporosis (see chapter 2, Who Is at Risk?).

But we still don't really know whether or not osteoporosis is becoming more common, because we don't have good historical records on osteoporosis in a large population. Today, doctors can precisely measure your bone mass, but until recently there was no way to diagnose osteoporosis in a living person until a bone broke. This means that a lot of osteoporosis probably went undetected.

Even so, osteoporosis is a serious problem affecting a growing number of people. The elderly population is projected to grow faster than the general population for the next several decades, as the baby boom generation reaches old age. Medical advances are making it possible for people to live longer, more active lives than ever before. Luckily, we are also learning more about the health of bone and how to protect it over the long term. Today, we can not only detect osteoporosis earlier; we can also treat it more effectively and with a wider range of conventional and alternative therapies than ever before.

Treating Osteoporosis: Medications and Natural Therapies

Today there are several conventional therapies that can prevent osteoporosis or keep it from getting worse. For women, the conventional therapies use estrogen or estrogen-like substances to offset the natural drop in the body's level of estrogen after menopause. Estrogen replacement therapy (ERT), hormone replacement therapy (HRT), and selective estrogen receptor modulators (SERMs) have all been shown to be effective against osteoporosis (we'll cover all three treatments in more detail later).

Another group of drugs known as *bisphosphonates* (including the drug alendronate) can actually build bone mass and thus reverse osteoporosis for both men and women. Each of these treatments has its advantages and disadvantages, and you should learn about all of them and discuss them with your doctor before making any decisions. See chapter 9, Conventional Treatments for Osteoporosis, for a description of these potentially life-saving therapies.

Yet medication is only part of the solution to a problem like osteoporosis. The medications mentioned previously usually can't be prescribed until relatively late in the game: at menopause for women, or at the actual onset of osteoporosis. Long before that point, you can be protecting yourself by making sure you're getting enough calcium, vitamin D, and other essential vitamins and minerals in your diet. Several nutritional supplements, especially calcium and vitamins D and K, may be used alone or in combination with medication to effectively treat osteoporosis by rebuilding weakened bones (see the chapters Calcium and Vitamin D for Osteoporosis and Other Important Nutrients for Your Bones). Your lifestyle and exercise habits are an important part of the picture as well (see chapter 7, Exercise, Diet, and Lifestyle: What You Can Do to Protect Your Bones).

Some highly promising treatments are called "natural" but are actually natural substances that have been slightly altered. Ipriflavone, a substance derived from soybeans that appears to mimic estrogen's effects on bone, may be as effective as estrogen therapy for osteoporosis—but with fewer side effects, and no estrogen effect anywhere else in the body. See chapter 5, Ipriflavone and Phytoestrogens, for a description of ipriflavone and other plant-based "natural" alternatives to estrogen therapy.

Who Is at Risk?

O steoporosis can strike anyone at any age, but some groups of people have higher rates of osteoporosis than others. The National Osteoporosis Foundation (www.nof.org) has identified eight factors that increase a person's risk for getting osteoporosis: age, gender, race, bone structure and body weight, menstrual history, lifestyle, medications and diseases, and family history.

If you have one or more of the risk factors described in this chapter, it doesn't necessarily mean you're going to get osteoporosis. Teenaged boys tend to have more car accidents than other people, but that doesn't mean *your* son will have an accident. It's certainly a good idea to discuss your risk factors with your doctor or health care provider, and to take sensible preventive measures like the ones described here. But don't panic—even if you do have several risk factors, there are many things you can do to protect your bones.

Likewise, it would be dangerous to assume you're *not* at risk simply because you don't have any of the risk factors discussed here. Individuals who don't have any known risk factors still get osteoporosis. For example, women as a group have a much higher risk than men, but significant numbers of men still get osteoporosis. Also, keep in mind that medical knowledge about this disease is growing, but far from perfect. There may be other risk factors that we simply don't know about yet.

Individuals who don't have any known risk factors still get osteoporosis.

Thanks to modern technology, you can learn whether you're at risk for osteoporotic fractures before they happen by having your bone density measured (see chapter 10, Evaluation and Screening for Osteoporosis).

Osteoporosis Risk Factors

Some risk factors can't be changed: your age and gender, for example, or your family history. Other factors you *can* change: your exercise, diet, and lifestyle habits.

Why learn about risk factors you can't change? Because if you take steps soon enough, osteoporotic fractures may be largely preventable. Even if you gain only a few years by evaluating your risk and getting an early diagnosis, you'll be much better off than if you'd simply waited for a fracture to occur. It's never too late to significantly reduce your risk of a fracture. Although you can't change your genes or your personal history, you'll be better able to decide about prevention and treatment options if you know your probable risk. Chapter 7, Exercise, Diet, and Lifestyle: What You Can Do to Protect Your Bones, discusses more fully how you can improve your odds.

Age

For both men and women, the risk for osteoporosis increases with age. After age 30 it's normal for both men and women to lose a small percentage of bone mass each year. In other words, the older you get, the more bone mass you lose.

Gender

Women are at much greater risk for osteoporosis than men. Of the 28 million people in the United States today who are at high risk for osteoporosis, 80% are women. In most countries in the Western world, women are twice as likely as men to fracture a hip.

Of the 28 million people in the United States today who are at high risk for osteoporosis, 80% are women.

This doesn't mean that men don't need to worry about osteoporosis. A significant number of men are affected as well—13% of white American men over age 50. In 1990, 30% of the 1.7 million hip fractures in the world occurred in men. Men are also more likely to die as a result of their hip fractures. Men are usually older when the fractures occur, and so they tend to have more serious complications as a result.[1]

Men lose bone mass as they get older, just as women do. But at every age, women are more likely than men to get osteoporosis. Women start out with less bone mineral density than men, and they may undergo a rapid period of bone loss for up to 6 years after menopause. Men lose only 20 to 30% of their bone mass during their lifetimes, while women may lose as much as 40 to 50%. Also,

Osteoporosis Risk Factors

The National Osteoporosis Foundation (www.nof.org) has identified eight factors that increase your risk of developing osteoporosis:

1. Age. The older you are, the greater your risk for osteoporosis.

2. Gender. Your chances of developing osteoporosis are greater if you are a woman.

3. Menstrual History. Normal or early menopause increases your risk of developing osteoporosis. Women who cease menstruating early because of disease, natural causes, eating disorders, or excessive exercise may be at higher risk for osteoporosis.

4. Race and Ancestry. Caucasian and Asian women are more likely to develop osteoporosis.

women tend to live longer than men, which means that there is more time for osteoporosis to progress.

Why do women have lower bone mineral density than men, even at peak bone mass? It may be because of hormonal factors, differences in men's and women's diets, or because most women in our society tend to do less intense exercise than men.[2] There is a great deal we don't know about the differences between the sexes when it comes to osteoporosis. Most of the research has focused on women. However, men do seem to benefit from the same changes in nutrition, exercise, and lifestyle that can help prevent osteoporosis in women.

5. Family History. Susceptibility to osteoporotic fractures may be, in part, hereditary. Young women whose mothers have a history of vertebral fractures also seem to have reduced bone mass.

6. Bone Structure and Body Weight. Small-boned and thin women are at greater risk.

7. Disease and Medications. Certain medications, including cortisone and related steroid drugs, increase your risk for osteoporosis. So do a number of diseases, including endocrine disorders, rheumatoid arthritis, and diseases that render you physically immobile.

8. Diet and Lifestyle. Smoking, excessive drinking, a diet low in calcium, and inadequate exercise all increase your risk for osteoporosis.

Menstrual History

As we've already seen, even normal menopause increases a woman's risk for osteoporosis by reducing her body's levels of the sex hormone *estrogen.* Likewise, if a woman's fertile (menstruating) years begin late or are cut short, her risk for osteoporosis may increase.

One study involving over 5,600 women throughout Europe found that women who began menstruating late (after the age of 15) were one and a half times more likely to fracture a hip after they turned 50. If they began menopause early (before the age of 44) they were 20% more likely to fracture a hip after 50 than if they had gone into menopause only 2 years later. In general, women who menstruated for at least 38 years were at lower risk than those whose menstruating life was shorter. And the longer a woman's fertile life was, the lower her risk for osteoporosis was found to be. Each additional fertile year past age 31 was associated with nearly a 2% decrease in the risk of a hip fracture.[3]

It is especially dangerous when young women stop menstruating. This can happen because of excessive exercise or eating disorders. The result can be rapid bone loss at an age when a woman should be building and maintaining her peak bone mass. Young women who do not menstruate can lose between 2% and 6% of their bone mass per year. A woman in her 20s could lose up to 25% of her bone mass, ending up with the bones of a 60-year-old before she turns 30.[4]

Chapter 3, Menopause, Estrogen, and Osteoporosis, discusses more fully the link between hormonal changes and osteoporosis.

Race and Ancestry

The ancient Greek historian Herodotus wrote that you could tell the nationality of a dead warrior by breaking his skull. Persian skulls were noticeably weak and easy to shatter, compared to the much harder skulls of Egyptians. This may be the first recorded observation of the link between bone density and genes.

Today we know that certain racial and ethnic groups have higher rates of osteoporotic fractures than others, because of differences in their bone mass. People of northern European (Caucasian) and Asian descent have lower average bone mass and higher rates of osteoporotic fractures than those whose ancestors came from Africa or the Mediterranean region.

This isn't to say that African-Americans don't have to worry about osteoporosis. People of all ancestries get osteoporosis. There is some intriguing evidence that African-American women may be at much higher risk for osteoporosis than South African women of African descent, suggesting that it's not safe to make broad assumptions about your risk for osteoporosis based on your ancestry.[5] According to one medical textbook author, genes account for only 70 to 80% of the acquisition of bone mass.[6]

Family History

Your family's genes also affect your bone size and thus your risk for osteoporosis. Small, thin people are at higher risk than large, muscular, big-boned people. If your older relatives have osteoporosis, your risk is higher. In fact, a family history of an osteoporotic fracture can increase your risk by one and one-half to three times the normal risk.

Remember, though, that no single factor absolutely determines your risk for osteoporosis. Genes are only part of a complex picture. In fact, in one study of perimenopausal women, researchers couldn't successfully predict who would get osteoporosis even after examining both genetic and environmental risk factors.[7]

Childhood Lifestyle

Bone is living tissue that grows when we use it in intense physical activity and nourish it with the right essential nutrients. Likewise, it's weakened by poor nutrition and physical immobility. But the most important time in your life for building strong bones is your childhood and teens, up until you reach your peak bone mass in your early 20s.

Studies have shown a connection between people's risk for osteoporosis and their level of physical activity and calcium intake during formative childhood years. It appears that the more physically active children are, and the higher their dietary calcium, the higher their peak bone mass will be—and there is a good chance that a high peak

Building Your Child's Peak Bone Mass

The first 20 years of life are the time when people are building peak bone mass. Make sure that your children and grandchildren are getting enough calcium and vitamin D in their diets. This is especially true for girls in their teens, a stage when many girls' calcium intake decreases. It's also important that children and teens are physically active and do weight-bearing exercise, such as running, jumping, bicycling, hiking, weight-lifting, racket sports, and cross-country skiing. It's been estimated that 75% of adolescents and young adults today do *not* have daily exercise. A sedentary childhood can increase your child's risk for osteoporosis as an adult.

bone mass will lower their risk for osteoporosis later in life.[8,9,10] See chapter 7, Exercise, Diet, and Lifestyle: What You Can Do to Protect Your Bones, for more information on which kinds of exercise are most helpful for building and maintaining bone mass.

Bone Structure and Body Weight

For both men and women, being thin increases the risk of getting osteoporosis. People who weigh more put more stress on their bones, and in response their bone mass tends to be higher.

There may be another reason why overweight women get osteoporosis less commonly. The sex hormone *estrogen* plays an important role in maintaining bone mass. After a woman goes through menopause, her body produces much less estrogen and progesterone than before. However, her body will continue to make small amounts of estrogen and progesterone from the adrenal glands. These glands will also produce testosterone (commonly thought of as a male sex hormone), although the amount appears to decrease with menopause. Adrenal androgens, hormones that come from the adrenal glands and can be made into estrogen, can be converted into estrone (an active form of estrogen) in the fat tissues in our bodies. Therefore, women with large stores of body fat can continue to produce much more estrogen after menopause than thin women can, and this may protect their bones.[11] Likewise, women who lose too much body fat (either through excessive exercise or eating disorders) may be at higher risk for osteoporosis.

Disease

There are many diseases and disorders that can reduce your bone mass. Alcoholism and anorexia nervosa, among other conditions, can harm your bones by robbing your body of essential nutrients. Stomach and digestive disorders such as Crohn's disease, celiac sprue, and inflammatory bowel disease may interfere with your body's ability to absorb calcium and other minerals. Certain cancers can directly harm bone, especially multiple myeloma (cancer of plasma cells in the bone marrow). Hyperthyroidism (an overactive thyroid gland) and Cushing's syndrome (a disorder of the adrenal gland) produce hormonal changes that cause bone to break down at an accelerated rate. Insulin-dependent diabetes and diseases of the liver and kidney (especially primary biliary cirrhosis) are other diseases that increase the risk of osteoporosis.

In women, the sex hormone estrogen plays an important role in protecting bone mass. Women who lose their ovaries through surgery, or undergo early menopause, face an increased risk for osteoporosis. The same is true for men with low testosterone levels.

Bones are also weakened by inactivity. Paralysis and immobility from strokes or other medical conditions can increase the risk of osteoporosis.[12]

Medications

Ironically, many modern medications—some of which literally save lives—also have a seriously detrimental side effect: they can greatly increase the risk that you'll get osteoporosis. We are not suggesting that you stop taking these medications if you need them. However, you should be aware of the risks involved, so that if you must take them you can also take extra preventive measures to protect your bones. If you are on one of these medications and have concerns about osteoporosis, discuss them with a doctor.

There is some evidence that taking calcium plus vitamin D may protect against bone loss induced by corticosteroids and possibly other medications. See chapter 4, Calcium and Vitamin D for Osteoporosis, for more information.

Corticosteroid Medications (Prednisone, Decadron, Dexamethasone, Prednisolone)

Corticosteroids are prescribed for a wide variety of illnesses, from rheumatoid arthritis to asthma. Although they can be very effective medications, if they're taken over a long period of time (more than a few months) they can cause a number of serious side effects, one of which is bone loss. Corticosteroids appear to pull a triple-whammy on your bones by decreasing your body's absorption of calcium, causing you to excrete more calcium in your urine, and inhibiting the function of the osteoblasts, the cells that form new bone. This effect is even worse for women who are postmenopausal; for them, even a small (7.5 mg daily) dosage of prednisone can cause bone loss.[13]

Inhaled steroids (such as beclomethasone, fluticasone, and budesonide), used to treat asthma, emphysema, and hay fever, are much safer than oral steroids. Nonetheless, researchers have voiced concern that they may cause bone loss and increase fracture risk when used in high dosages for a long period of time.[14]

If you have concerns about your medication, please remember: it's never a good idea to stop taking corticosteroids abruptly or without your doctor's advice.

Thyroid Medications (Levothroid, Synthroid, Cytomel, Euthyroid, Thyrolar)

These medications are forms of thyroid hormone, usually prescribed for various conditions in which the thyroid gland produces too little of its own natural hormone. The thyroid gland plays an important role in regulating the formation of new bone. Unfortunately, if you get too much thyroid hormone it can increase your risk for osteoporosis. In chapter 1 we described the osteoclasts, the cells that break down tiny particles of bone in the natural cycle of bone remodeling. An excess of thyroid hormone can stimulate the osteoclasts to break down too much bone.

This potential side effect of thyroid medication isn't as great a problem today as it used to be, because doctors can now monitor a patient's level of thyroid-stimulating hormone (TSH) in the blood. This test allows doctors to make sure their patients aren't getting too much thyroid medication. TSH monitoring isn't foolproof, but it's much safer than taking thyroid medications without it. If you have concerns about a thyroid medication, please discuss them with your doctor, and remember: never stop taking thyroid medication abruptly, or without a doctor's advice.

Depo-Provera (Medroxyprogesterone Acetate)

Depo-Provera is used most commonly as an injection or implant to prevent pregnancy. It is also used to treat excessive uterine bleeding. Depo-Provera is a long-acting progestin, a laboratory-produced variation of the sex hormone progesterone. Depo-Provera is known to significantly increase the risk of osteoporosis.[15]

One study published in the *British Medical Journal* revealed that women who were long-term users of Depo-Provera experienced an average loss of 7.5% bone density in the spine.[16] On a positive note, the same researchers looked at whether bone loss occurring in women using Depo-Provera could be reversed once the medication was stopped. In a follow-up study, they found that women who stopped using depot medroxyprogesterone (an equivalent to Depo-Provera) experienced a mean increase of 6.4% in their lumbar spine bone density after two years. Although the women didn't gain bone density back in their hips, they were at least able to maintain the level of bone density there.[17]

Because Depo-Provera can offer benefits as well, it is advisable to discuss the pros and cons of taking it with your physician.

Gonadotropin-Releasing Hormone Agonists (GnRH Agonists)

These medications are sometimes used to treat reproductive disorders such as endometriosis, uterine fibroids, and polycystic ovaries (in women) and prostate cancer (in men). In women, they shut down the ovaries and dramatically lower the body's level of estrogen. Research has shown bone loss in women taking these drugs for 6 months or longer.[18]

Other Medications

Other types of medications that may increase your risk for bone loss and osteoporosis are:

- Chemotherapy
- Lithium

- Anticonvulsants (Tegretol, Dilantin, Depakote, Pheno-barbital)
- Immunosuppressive agents used in organ transplants (Cyclosporin A)
- Heparin
- Isoniazid
- Tamoxifen (in premenopausal women only)[19,20]

If you are taking one of these medications, you and your doctor should discuss your risk for osteoporosis.

The following medications may present an increased risk of osteoporosis. None of them has been shown directly to cause bone loss in human beings. But some have been found to be toxic to bone in animal studies, and others might have a negative effect on calcium metabolism in humans:

- Long-term tetracycline use
- Diuretics that increase calcium in the urine (Lasix)
- Aluminum-containing antacids (Rolaids, Di-Gel, Gaviscon, Maalox, Mylanta)

Diet and Lifestyle

Even in adulthood, your exercise habits, use of alcohol and tobacco, and intake of calcium can influence your risk for osteoporosis. The following sections briefly discuss certain diet and lifestyle risk factors. Chapter 7, Exercise, Diet, and Lifestyle: What You Can Do to Protect Your Bones, describes in greater detail some of the lifestyle changes you might want to consider if you're concerned about your risk for osteoporosis.

Alcohol

Does drinking alcohol increase your risk for osteoporosis? It depends. There is some evidence suggesting that alcohol poisons osteoblasts, the cells responsible for building new bone.[21,22] However, studies suggest that the amount of alcohol consumed may be an important factor in determining how alcohol affects bone.

One 12-year observational study actually found that postmenopausal women who drank moderately had a lower rate of postmenopausal bone loss.[23] Another study showed an association between moderate alcohol consumption and higher bone mineral density in women and men, as well.[24] However, since people who drink in moderation may also have other healthy lifestyle habits that could affect their bone mass, it's not clear that there's a direct cause-and-effect relationship between alcohol and bone mass.

Excessive drinking, on the other hand, does seem to have a negative effect. Research has found that people who consume large quantities of alcohol daily have an increased risk of fractures and lower bone mass. It's not clear whether this is because alcohol directly harms bone, but some of the chemicals responsible for osteoporosis in women with low estrogen levels are also present in individuals who have alcohol-related liver disease.[25] Heavy drinking also increases the risk of falling, which of course often leads to broken bones.

Smoking (Tobacco)

Studies also suggest (though not consistently) that smokers have a higher risk for osteoporosis than nonsmokers. One reason may be related to the effect that tobacco smoke has on the metabolism of estrogen and other hormones. (In men, too, smoking changes the metabolism of sex hormones). Women who smoke enter menopause about 2 years earlier than non smoking women, have higher rates of vertebral fractures, and have lower bone mass after entering menopause.[26,27] Postmenopausal women who smoke lose more bone mass than postmenopausal women who are nonsmokers.[28,29] Male smokers, too, are at higher risk for osteoporosis. In a 16-year study of male smokers compared to nonsmokers, one-pack-per-day smokers lost bone mass at nearly *twice* the rate of nonsmokers. Smoking was found to be a significant risk factor for bone loss in men who smoked more than 10 cigarettes a day.[30]

Diet

It will come as no surprise that your bones are better off when you get enough calcium in your diet. Your bones are largely made of calcium. Other systems in your body also need calcium to function. If your diet doesn't supply enough, your body may break down bone tissue to release calcium into your blood for other uses. Chapter 4, Calcium and Vitamin D for Osteoporosis, explains how much calcium you need for optimal health, as well as the many different sources of dietary calcium.

You also need an adequate amount of vitamin D in your body to absorb and use calcium to make bone. Chapter 4 describes more fully the sources of vitamin D and the recommended dosages.

For many years it has been believed that excess protein also increases the risk for bone loss. When our bodies get too much protein, we excrete what we don't need in the form of urinary nitrogen, and the laws of chemistry cause calcium to go out along with it. Based on this observation, as well as other evidence, experts concluded that excessive protein was a risk factor for osteoporosis.[31,32] The average recommended daily intake is 50 g for women and 63 g for men, but the American average is closer to 95 g, most of it coming from meat and dairy products. But other research seems to suggest otherwise.[33]

A recent observational study, the Iowa Women's Health Study, found that groups of women who had lower protein intakes, especially those under 49 g of protein a day, had higher percentages of hip fractures when compared to those eating more than 70 g per day.[34] The actual number of women in the study who had hip fractures was small, however: 44 women out of 32,006. Therefore, it's not clear whether this is a meaningful result or a statistical fluke. So what's the bottom line? At present, we can't tell you for certain whether eating excessive protein is bad for your bones. Consult your health care provider for advice.

Excessive sodium can also cause you to lose calcium in the urine.

Excessive sodium can also cause you to lose calcium in the urine. In the United States, most of us eat too much sodium in the form of *sodium chloride* (table salt). Processed foods such as cheese, lunch meats, crackers, and snack foods such as potato chips, pickles, olives, and salsa are often very high in sodium. In fact, in one study, researchers determined that postmenopausal women would need to take 1,000 mg of dietary calcium each day to prevent the bone loss that occurs at the hip from consuming 2,000 mg of sodium daily.[35,36] While 2,000 mg may seem like a lot of salt to take in, it's not hard to do if you regularly eat processed foods!

Caffeine is often mentioned as a possible risk factor in osteoporosis, but the evidence is conflicting. Caffeine is an alkaloid found in coffee, tea, chocolate, and cola soft drinks. It is a *diuretic,* meaning that it causes increased urination, although this effect tends to decrease with continued use.

Caffeine causes calcium to be secreted in the urine. For example, one study of 170 premenopausal women found that a small intake of caffeine was associated with a higher loss of calcium in the urine.[37] In addition, the 12-year-long Framingham study of 3,170 women found that women who drank more than 2 1/2 cups of coffee per day had an increased risk for osteoporotic fractures.[38]

However, other studies have failed to identify such a connection, and still others have found evidence that drinking caffeinated tea may actually decrease a woman's risk for fracture.[39] Despite the lack of scientific clarity on this issue, since excessive caffeine isn't good for you for other health reasons as well, it is probably wise to limit yourself to a moderate amount of coffee, chocolate, and other sources of caffeine.

Regular, moderate exercise to suit your age and ability level is one of the most important things you can do to protect yourself from osteoporosis.

Exercise

Like muscle, bone becomes stronger when you use it and weaker when you don't. Bed rest can cause a person to lose bone very rapidly, by as much as 1% of total bone mass *per week*. Regular, moderate exercise to suit your age and ability level is one of the most important things you can do to protect yourself from osteoporosis. Chapter 7, Exercise, Diet, and Lifestyle: What You Can Do to Protect Your Bones, describes several recommended types of exercise for protecting your bones.

Menopause, Estrogen, and Osteoporosis

I t's natural for everyone to lose a little bone mass (perhaps 1 to 2%) each year after age 65 or so. But women may lose a good deal more bone mass in the years immediately following menopause. For about 3 to 6 years after menopause, a woman may lose as much as 5% or more of her total bone mass each year. At the end of this period, she may have lost as much as 25 to 30% of her total bone mass. This loss of bone mass following menopause is clearly a major cause in many cases of osteoporosis in postmenopausal women.[1]

You may already know that one of the leading ways to help prevent osteoporosis is for women to take supplemental estrogen after menopause. Some conventional and alternative treatments work by imitating estrogen's helpful effects. The following sections illustrate the relationship between estrogen, menopause, and your bones.

How Estrogen Protects Your Bones

Why does such rapid bone loss occur after menopause? The major reason seems to be a decline in the body's levels of *estrogen,* the female sex hormone. Estrogen protects women's bones by inhibiting the activity of *osteoclasts,* the cells that break down and resorb bone.[2,3]

Our bodies are continually carrying out a natural cycle of bone remodeling, in which old, stressed bone tissue is destroyed and new bone cells are created. As long as there is a balance between both halves of this cycle—destruction and creation—bone remodeling serves us well. Estrogen plays an important role in maintaining the balance. But when your body begins to produce less estrogen after menopause, the destruction half of the cycle can outpace the creation of new bone, and the result is a significant net loss of bone each year.

When your body begins to produce less estrogen after menopause, the destruction half of the cycle can outpace the creation of new bone, and the result is a significant net loss of bone each year.

Menopause

When a woman goes through menopause, the various mechanisms in her body that have made her fertile begin to change. Primarily, her body produces much less estrogen. Before menopause, most of the body's estrogen is produced by the ovaries, which also make another important sex hormone: progesterone. Progesterone may play a role in osteoporosis as well.

After menopause, the ovaries' production of these hormones drops to a very low level. Small amounts of estrogen and progesterone continue to be made in other parts of the body, but the levels of both hormones remain permanently much lower after menopause.

Other Causes of Estrogen Loss

A woman's estrogen levels can decline for reasons other than natural menopause. Younger women who cease menstruating for other reasons—for example, because of eating disorders or overly intensive exercise regimens—may suffer permanent loss of bone.[4]

Surgical Removal of the Ovaries (Bilateral Oophorectomy)

Sometimes, because of disease or other reasons, a woman's ovaries have to be surgically removed. Because the ovaries produce most of the body's sex hormones until menopause, this type of surgery permanently reduces the body's levels of estrogen as well as progesterone. Usually, a woman who has had this surgery would be prescribed estrogen, with or without a form of progesterone. However, there are some health risks associated with taking supplemental hormones, and women with certain health conditions can't take them. Without supplemental hormone therapy, surgical removal of the ovaries greatly increases the risk for osteoporosis.

Late Menarche or Early Menopause

Some women simply have shorter fertile lives than others, either because they begin menstruating later than most girls, or because menopause comes early. In either case, a shorter menstrual life means fewer years of estrogen protecting the bones, and thus a higher eventual risk for bone loss and osteoporosis.

Exercise and Amenorrhea (Lack of Menstrual Periods)

Although exercise is generally good for your bones, sometimes women train so strenuously that they stop menstruating, at least temporarily. Some research has indicated that among premenopausal, highly skilled and trained female athletes, 15% of runners and 28% of gymnasts have ceased menstruating. Where this is the case, the risk for osteoporosis is much higher.

Strenuous exercise is very helpful for strengthening the bones. But if you exercise enough to stop your period, the negative effects outweigh the gain. Young women who do not menstruate can lose bone mass rapidly— from 2 to 6% of total bone mass

Strenuous exercise is very helpful for strengthening the bones. But if you exercise enough to stop your period, the negative effects outweigh the gain.

each year. And the consequences are doubly serious for a young woman who loses bone when she should be building and maintaining her peak bone mass. A young female athlete in her 20s who experiences amenorrhea from intensive exercise could lose up to 25% of her total bone mass in a few years, placing her at great risk for osteoporotic fractures in later years.[5] Beyond this long-term risk, the risk for fractures is even more immediate. In one study of female ballet dancers, researchers found that stress fractures were similarly linked to both amenorrhea and heavy training. [6]

What Causes Women Athletes to Stop Menstruating?

Why do some women who do strenuous exercise stop having menstrual periods? A decrease may occur in the level of a brain hormone called gonadotropin-releasing hormone, which controls levels of estrogen and progesterone in the body. Many female athletes exercise to the extent that their bodies, in need of more energy, break down body fat stores. Women rely on fat stores to help produce estrogen, and once they lose too much body fat, the resulting lack of estrogen causes them to stop menstruating.

In addition, health risks are compounded when an athlete has anorexia nervosa, or any other eating disorder that results in a serious loss of body fat. And this is not a rare problem: studies have found that as many as 62% of female athletes in certain sports may develop eating disorders.[7]

Eating Disorders (Anorexia Nervosa)

Eating disorders such as anorexia affect a woman both hormonally and nutritionally. If a woman isn't taking in enough food, she'll tend to burn up her body's fat stores for energy. If these fat stores diminish too far, she may become unable to produce normal amounts of estrogen, because a woman's body depends on fat cells for some of its estrogen requirements. The result can be a rapid loss of bone that may not be regained even after the woman recovers from anorexia nervosa.[8]

Eating disorders such as anorexia or bulimia also prevent a woman from getting the calcium and other nutrients she needs to build and maintain healthy bones.

Other Causes of Amenorrhea

Medications that suppress the body's production of estrogen (e.g., Provera and GnRH agonists) can have a similarly harmful effect on bone.

Therapies That Replace or Mimic Estrogen

If a loss of estrogen leads to osteoporosis, can't you prevent osteoporosis by boosting your body's levels of estrogen? The answer is yes. The leading medical therapy to prevent osteoporosis in postmenopausal women is called estrogen replacement therapy (ERT). In ERT, a woman takes a synthetic or animal- or plant-derived estrogen to replace what her body once made naturally. Often, the estrogen is combined with a progestin, a chemical cousin of the sex hormone progesterone, to counter the increased risk for uterine cancer that occurs when estrogen is taken alone. The term used to describe the combination of estrogen with a progestin is hormone replacement therapy (HRT).

For preventing osteoporosis, HRT is clearly effective, especially with long-term use (5 or more years).[9] With either natural or surgically induced menopause, HRT prevents or at least delays bone loss in the majority of the women who take it.[10] Estrogen doesn't prevent normal age-related bone loss, which happens in both men and women as their bodies become less able to absorb calcium, but it does effectively protect women against the potentially devastating rapid loss of bone that occurs in the early years of menopause.

However, estrogen comes with certain risks and disadvantages. Taken alone, estrogen (as ERT) greatly increases a woman's risk for cancer of the uterine lining (endometrium). As mentioned previously, this risk of uterine cancer is typically minimized by combining estrogen with a progestin (HRT).

But there is also some evidence that taking supplemental estrogen may increase your risk for certain types of breast cancer, especially if you take estrogen in high doses or for more than 5 years. Yet it's only after 5 or more years that estrogen seems to be most effective in preventing bone loss. Furthermore, if you stop taking estrogen at any point after menopause, you begin to lose bone again—which generally means that you have to take estrogen over the long term to get its bone-protecting benefits. And taking a progestin will not protect you from this risk of breast cancer. In fact, two recent studies give reasonably strong evidence that the use of estrogen and progestins together (HRT) may put women at a substantially higher risk for breast cancer than use of estrogen (ERT) alone.[11,12] In addition, many women prefer not to take ERT or HRT for reasons other than their concerns about breast cancer.

Two recent studies give reasonably strong evidence that the use of estrogen and progestins together (HRT) may put women at a substantially higher risk for breast cancer than use of estrogen (ERT) alone.

While many doctors believe that the benefits of ERT and HRT still outweigh their risks for most women, these therapies are uniformly not prescribed in two specific cases: Estrogen cannot be given to a woman who has breast cancer, or who has ever had it in the past. Research has shown that estrogen can dramatically speed up the

Lorna's Story

Lorna, a 45-year-old breast cancer survivor, no longer menstruated as a result of her cancer treatment. She knew her early medically induced "menopause" might increase her risk for osteoporosis, but she was determined to stay healthy. When she was first diagnosed with cancer, she immediately gave up cigarettes and alcohol, started to eat a healthier diet, and began a regular exercise program. Lorna was clearly willing to make changes in her lifestyle for the sake of her health.

Because of her breast cancer, estrogen replacement therapy wasn't an option for Lorna. Yet in addition to her loss of menstruation, she had other risk factors for osteoporosis: She was thin and small-boned, and she had smoked for several years. A bone scan revealed that she had low bone mass (osteopenia), a condition that can lead to osteoporosis. Aside from taking hormones, what could she do to protect her bones?

Her doctor had good news for Lorna: she had a number of options. Many medications, natural supplements, and dietary and lifestyle changes can help decrease your risk for osteoporosis even if your levels of estrogen are low.

progression of breast cancer and also increase the chance of a recurrence after successful treatment.

The findings mentioned here obviously have important ramifications regarding the use of both ERT and HRT. You'll find them discussed more fully in chapter 9, Conventional Treatments for Osteoporosis, along with the pros and cons of a relatively new generation of drugs, *selective estrogen receptor modulators,* designed to deliver estrogen's positive bone-protecting effects with none of its troublesome ones. In the meantime, if you are currently using ERT or HRT and have questions about the impact of these therapies on your health, we strongly encourage you not to discontinue them on your own. Speak with your health care provider to determine what regimen might best suit your health needs and concerns.

Ipriflavone

You may be aware that natural estrogen-like substances present in soybeans and other plants (phytoestrogens) may be helpful in easing some symptoms of menopause like hot flashes. (Visit us on the Web at www.TNP.com for more information.)

However, there is also a dietary supplement derived from naturally occurring compounds found in soybeans that mimics estrogen's positive effects on bone: ipriflavone. Ipriflavone has been studied extensively enough to give us meaningful evidence of its effectiveness. (See chapter 5, Ipriflavone and Phytoestrogens, for more detail.) Like estrogen, ipriflavone appears to restrict the osteoclasts from breaking down too much bone tissue in the bone remodeling cycle. While it has estrogen-like effects in the body that target the bone, ipriflavone appears to be completely free of any estrogen-like activity as far as the breast and uterus are concerned.

Ipriflavone has another potential advantage: If combined with ERT, it seems to enhance estrogen's bone-protecting effects. For example, one study looked at whether ipriflavone combined with a normal dosage of estrogen (.625 mg oral conjugated estrogens daily) could prevent the rapid bone loss that occurs in women whose ovaries have been surgically removed. It found that when taken together, ipriflavone plus estrogen stopped bone loss in these women, something that neither therapy taken by itself could do.[13] Some evidence also suggests that a combination of ipriflavone and a low dosage of estrogen may protect bone as well as, or even better than, a normal dose of estrogen.[14] This is an exciting finding, as it suggests a way that women might be able to reduce their dosage of estrogen (and thus its side effects and health risks) without sacrificing any protection against osteoporosis.

However, we need more research to establish whether it's safe to combine ipriflavone and estrogen in this way. At least one animal study suggests that ipriflavone might enhance estrogen's effect on the uterine lining as well as on bone when these therapies are taken together.[15] This might mean that ipriflavone would enhance the risk of endometrial cancer, and perhaps other health risks associated with estrogen replacement therapy.

While it has estrogen-like effects in the body that target the bone, ipriflavone appears to be completely free of any estrogen-like activity as far as the breast and uterus are concerned.

Until more evidence is available, we can't recommend that you combine ipriflavone with estrogen replacement therapy except under the close supervision of a qualified health care professional. Another approach might be to combine vitamin D and calcium supplements with a low dosage of estrogen. These combination treatments might eliminate some of the health risks involved in taking estrogen, by cutting the dosage in half. For more information see chapters 4 and 5.

Calcium and Vitamin D for Osteoporosis

O ne of the safest, least expensive ways to protect yourself against osteoporosis is to add a calcium supplement of 500 mg to 1,000 mg daily to your routine. Calcium can be safely combined with hormone replacement therapy or any other osteoporosis treatment you may be using. And it's even more effective when you take vitamin D with your calcium. Scientific studies have shown calcium to be effective in slowing or stopping bone loss. When vitamin D is added, these two nutrients can even rebuild weakened bone and significantly reduce your risk for a fracture. Together, they can enhance the bone-protecting effectiveness of hormone replacement therapy and other medications.

Your bones are made of calcium crystals, collagen, and other minerals. An adult skeleton contains roughly 1 to 2 kg of calcium, all of which originally entered the body through food or other external sources. All your life, you need a steady supply of calcium to build new bone and support other vital functions.

It should be no surprise that the amount of calcium you get in your diet is important for the health of your bones. But, as we will see, most Americans don't get enough calcium. If your diet provides too little calcium, your body will *resorb* some bone tissue to release calcium back into the bloodstream. The net effect is that inadequate calcium intake contributes to bone weakness.

Calcium can be safely combined with hormone replacement therapy or any other osteoporosis treatment you may be using.

Another important factor is vitamin D. Without an adequate amount of this vitamin, your body can't effectively absorb and use calcium to build bone. This section describes how these two important nutrients can help you prevent and treat osteoporosis at all stages in life.

How Much Calcium Do You Need?

It is thought that our Paleolithic ancestors ate about 1,500 mg of calcium daily, which would put them well ahead of us today.[1] Even higher calcium intake has been reported for some of the world's few remaining hunter-gatherer tribes: 2,100 to 3,000 mg each day or more.[2] (Interestingly, these hunter-gatherers eat no milk or cheese. They get much of their calcium from plant-based foods.)

Today we get far less calcium than our ancestors did. The average daily calcium intake of a postmenopausal woman in the United States is only 600 mg. At least 90% of young children, adult women, teenaged girls, and adult men get less than the recommended daily intake (see table 2, Recommended Calcium Intakes). Even teenaged boys, who have the nation's highest calcium intake, generally get less than they should.[3]

One reason calcium deficiency is so common is that it's hard to get all the calcium you need from a modern diet. To get 1,000 mg of calcium (a typical daily recommendation), you'd have to drink about a quart of milk, or eat a quarter-pound of cheddar cheese or several healthy servings of kale or collard greens (see table 1, Good Food Sources of Calcium). For most of us, taking a supplement or a calcium-fortified food is the only practical way to get all the calcium we need.

Calcium Supplementation and Osteoporosis: The Evidence

What happens if your intake of calcium isn't high enough to meet your body's needs? In order to maintain adequate blood levels of calcium, your body will resorb extra bone. Clearly, it's better to avoid such withdrawals from the "calcium bank" of your bones. It is important to get enough calcium at all stages of life.

As you'll see, the research suggests that calcium works much more effectively when combined with vitamin D. (See chapter 6, Other Important Nutrients for Your Bones, for more information.) But even taken by itself, calcium can significantly slow bone loss in the elderly (it appears to do this in every part of the body except the spine). It may also be the key to the ultimate in prevention: building healthy, strong bones in children and adolescents.

Osteoporosis: A "Pediatric Disease"?

Though the symptoms of osteoporosis usually don't appear until late in life, some experts consider it a "pediatric disease" because, they argue, adequate amounts of calcium and exercise in childhood could go a long way toward preventing it. Remember that osteoporosis is strongly influ-

Table 1. Good Food Sources of Calcium[4,5,6]

Source (mg)	Serving Size	Calcium
DAIRY		
Milk, whole	1 cup	290
Milk, lowfat, 2%	1 cup	300
Cottage cheese	1 cup	130
Cheese, jack	1 oz	212
Yogurt, lowfat plain	1 cup	415
Yogurt, whole milk	1 cup	275
FISH		
Sardines, canned (with bones)	3 oz	372
Salmon, canned (with bones)	4 oz	90
Oysters	4 oz	107
VEGETABLES		
Kale	½ cup	74
Broccoli	½ cup	68
Collard greens	½ cup	105
Mustard greens	½ cup	97
BEANS		
Black-eyed peas	½ cup	106
Tofu (calcium-set)	½ cup	155
Soymilk (calcium-fortified)	1 cup	150–300
Hummus	½ cup	62
GRAINS		
Amaranth, boiled	1 cup	276
Teff, boiled	1 cup	200

enced by two things: your peak bone mass, and the rate at which you lose bone mass each year. And since peak bone mass is reached by age 20 or so, the best time to work on maximizing it is adolescence—or even earlier.

There is evidence that taking calcium supplements in childhood may increase peak bone mass, while inadequate calcium intake may slow the growth of bone.[7] One study in adolescent women found that calcium supplementation of 500 mg a day for 18 months increased several measurements of total body bone gain.[8] Though the gains reported in this study were relatively modest, their long-term significance cannot be underestimated: One clinical trial found that a 6% difference in the peak bone mass of two adult populations resulted in a large difference in hip fracture rates between these two groups.[9]

There is evidence that taking calcium supplements in childhood may increase peak bone mass, while inadequate calcium intake may slow the growth of bone.

Another study found that, by age 16, young women had already reached 90 to 97% of their mothers' premenopausal bone density.[10] While we don't know the precise age when peak bone mass is attained, this study suggests that the early to mid teens are a critical time in bone formation.

In one study reported in the _Journal of the American Medical Association,_ 11- and 12–year-old girls were given either 500 mg of calcium or placebo daily. ("Placebo" means a medically inactive substance such as a sugar pill.) The girls stayed on this regimen for 18 months while they ate a diet containing about 960 mg of calcium each day. At the end of the 18 months, several different bone mineral density measurements were taken. The girls who received calcium supplements had significantly better results than the placebo group. On average, the girls in the calcium group had gained an additional 1.3% of total bone mass

When Is the Best Time to Give Your Child Calcium?

A carefully designed study on 70 pairs of identical twins, ages 6 to 14, provided strong evidence for giving children calcium *before puberty.* Over 3 years, one twin from each pair took a supplement of 700 mg of calcium citrate malate each day. The other twin received no supplemental calcium. After 3 years, it was found that the calcium made a significant difference in the bone mass of children who hadn't gone through puberty yet. But the older children did *not* get a significant benefit from taking the calcium.[13]

per year. Such an increase is large enough to make a real difference in even a few years.[11]

Other research found similar results. In one study of 112 girls aged 11 and 12, girls who took a supplement of 500 mg of calcium daily for two years gained an additional 1.5% of their total bone mass *each year,* compared to the placebo group.[12]

Calcium Later in Life Slows or Even Stops Bone Loss

In 1990, researchers pulled together the results of 49 separate studies involving calcium supplements and bone mass.[14] Although not all studies had the same results, in general the research showed that calcium supplements reduced bone loss in postmenopausal women in every bone site measured except the spine. Twelve of the 49 studies analyzed were double-blind placebo-controlled trials—the best type of study for eliminating the power of suggestion and proving that a treatment really is effective. Six of these well-designed studies involved women in their 50s

The Placebo Effect

Doctors have long known that people tend to feel somewhat better after they take a pill they *believe* will help them—even if it's only a sugar pill. How do you know if a treatment is effective? One way is to compare its effects to those of a placebo—a medically inactive, harmless substance such as a sugar pill. If the treatment works better than placebo, then it must be truly effective. A placebo-controlled study is one in which a treatment is compared against a placebo. Because the placebo effect only works if there is genuine belief, such studies should also be double-blinded, meaning that neither researchers nor subjects know exactly who is getting the treatment and who is only getting placebo.

who were not taking estrogen replacement therapy or any medication to prevent bone loss. The results of all six studies were very consistent. Although calcium supplements reduced these women's bone loss by an amount that equaled 0.8% of total bone mass per year, on average, its protective effects were not observed in the spine, or for women in the immediate postmenopausal years. This suggests that calcium alone probably isn't enough to protect a woman against the rapid bone loss that often comes in the 3 to 6 years following menopause—but it helps.

In general, calcium supplements seemed to be most effective in women who were older, already had osteoporosis, and had a history of low calcium intake.

A 1990 study of 301 women who had never used estrogen found even more dramatic results: evidence that calcium supplements (500 mg daily) could actually *stop* bone loss in the hips and arms of postmenopausal women.[15] But this double-blind placebo-controlled study suggested that calcium supplements might work better for compact rather than spongy (trabecular) bone. The calcium supplementation did *not* protect these women against losing spinal bone. They lost an average of 1% per year—enough to eventually lead to osteoporosis for many women. (Spinal bone is mostly trabecular.)

A study published in 1995 observed the long-term effects of a higher dosage of calcium on bone loss and fractures in postmenopausal women. In this double-blind placebo-controlled study, 86 women previously enrolled in a two year clinical trial by these same researchers agreed to continue on with either a higher daily dosage of calcium (1,000 mg of elemental calcium in the form of 5.24 g of calcium lactate/gluconate and 800 mg of calcium carbonate) or

Although not all studies had the same results, in general the research showed that calcium supplements reduced bone loss in postmenopausal women in every bone site measured except the spine.

placebo. The women were all at least 3 years past menopause, and their average age was 58. Their diets contained an average of about 670 mg of calcium a day as well. The results were promising. During the 4 years of the study, the women's bone density was measured at various sites, including the spine. In those who took calcium, bone loss in the spine was reduced in the group taking calcium during the first year of the study, but not subsequently. Over the entire study period, however, women who took calcium lost

The Milk Puzzle

Although milk had been considered a good source of calcium, recent research suggests that women who drink more milk may be *more* likely to break a bone. A study published in the *American Journal of Public Health* in 1997 looked at long-term effects of milk on bone density. The study followed 77,761 nurses (ages 34 to 59) for 12 years, looking at the amount of milk in their diets and the number of hip and wrist fractures they suffered during that time. The women who reported drinking two or more glasses of milk every day had a risk for hip fracture that was approximately one and a half times greater than women who drank one glass or less.[17] None of these women were taking calcium pills, and the researchers carefully ruled out the idea that other factors such as exercise, smoking, or medications could explain this puzzling result, which seems to contradict common sense. After all, research has shown that calcium is good for your bones, and we know that milk is a good source of calcium—right?

less bone in the spine compared to those taking placebo. Similarly, the greatest benefit of calcium in the hip was also noted to be during year one. However, women who took calcium had significantly less total body bone mineral density loss over the 4-year study's duration. Given these positive effects on bone mineral density, the researchers concluded that if the women continued to take calcium supplementation over a 30-year period during their postmenopausal lives, the cumulative benefits would be enough to potentially cut their risk of a fracture by half.[16]

Given these surprising results, the researchers spent time postulating possible explanations for the increased risk for hip fracture in women consuming greater amounts of dairy foods. They concluded that it was most likely due to some other characteristic of the women who ate the dairy foods or to some other nutrient or non-nutrient component of the dairy foods, rather than to the dairy calcium itself. For example, milk contains other minerals that can reduce the helpful effect of the calcium. Too much phosphorus can reduce your ability to benefit from calcium in your diet. Some researchers have theorized that the phosphorus content of milk makes the calcium less absorbable, but we don't really know. It's also possible that the milk drinkers in the study ate more sodium than the other women, or had some other, unidentified habits that reduced their ability to use calcium from the milk they drank. What the study does point out is that calcium from dairy products alone may not protect you from fracturing a bone.

Vitamin D: Calcium's Partner in Building Bone

Vitamin D is actually considered a hormone. Though we can get it from foods (fish oil, butter, eggs, and fortified milk), our bodies make as much as 80 to 90% of the vitamin D we use. To make vitamin D, we need about 15 minutes a day of direct sunlight on our skin. Our bodies use sunlight to convert certain precursor chemicals into usable vitamin D.

Today, many North Americans and Europeans are at risk for vitamin D deficiency. Why? Many of us spend too much time indoors to get enough direct sunlight, and when we use sunblock to protect ourselves against skin cancer, we also reduce our production of vitamin D. Furthermore, in northern parts of the United States and throughout Canada, the angle of sunlight in winter doesn't allow enough ultraviolet rays to reach people from October to March. Additionally, as we get older it's harder for our skin to produce vitamin D, and so deficiencies are more common in people over 60.[18] Age also reduces our ability to make the active form of vitamin D in our kidneys.

Many North Americans and Europeans are at risk for vitamin D deficiency.

How common is vitamin D deficiency? In healthy, non-hospitalized people, deficiencies have been found in 14% of women and 6% of men. But among people in hospitals, one study found deficiencies in 57% of patients.[19] And among residents in their 80s living in nursing homes in the Netherlands (mostly women), 79% were found to have vitamin D deficiencies.

Since our bodies need vitamin D in order to use calcium for building bone, it would seem logical to take vitamin D supplements in addition to calcium. In fact, the scientific research shows clearly that calcium supplements are much more effective against osteoporosis when they're taken with vitamin D as well.

Vitamin D with Calcium: The Evidence

Calcium supplements taken alone can slow or even possibly stop bone loss, especially in compact rather than spongy bone—that is, in the hips and wrists rather than in the spine. But when you combine calcium with vitamin D, the benefits are even more dramatic. One recent commentary in *The New England Journal of Medicine* mentioned three landmark studies which showed that taking calcium with vitamin D can not only protect against bone loss, but can actually rebuild bone.[20]

The first study involved 249 women in Boston, where the winter sunlight is too scanty to provide enough vitamin D. These women, whose average age was 61, were all postmenopausal, and none were taking estrogen or any medication to prevent bone loss. Half the women received placebo and the other half received a vitamin D supplement of 400 IU daily. In addition, women in both groups received about 400 mg of calcium citrate malate daily. Both groups of women also had some calcium and vitamin D (about 100 IU) in their

Taking calcium with vitamin D can not only protect against bone loss, but can actually rebuild bone.

diets. After 1 year, the women's bone density was measured. The results were impressive: the women who took supplemental calcium and vitamin D actually *gained* spinal bone mass (0.85%).[21] Again, the spine, which is mostly made of spongy (trabecular) bone, is the one place that responded least to calcium supplementation alone.

A second study found more modest results after 3 years on a regimen of 500 mg calcium citrate malate and 700 IU vitamin D daily. This study, which enrolled men and women over age 65, found that the group receiving treatment had moderately reduced bone loss in the hip, spine, and total body compared to the placebo group over the 3-year period. (None of the women were receiving estrogen or any other medication to prevent bone loss). In

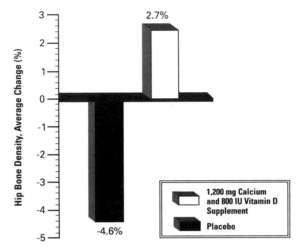

Figure 5. *Placebo vs. calcium/vitamin D supplement in women*

addition, the study participants who took calcium and vitamin D had 50% fewer non-spinal fractures than did those in the placebo group.[22]

A large French study examined whether vitamin D plus calcium would have the same effect on compact (cortical) bone. The study participants (3,270 women aged 78 to 90 years) were split into two groups. One group took placebo, and the other received a daily supplement of 1,200 mg of calcium and 800 IU vitamin D. After 18 months of this regimen, the women's bone density was measured. The placebo group had experienced an average decrease of 4.6% in their hip bone density. But the women who'd taken vitamin D and calcium had an average *increase* of 2.7% (see figure 5). During the 18 months of the study, the women taking the supplements had 43% fewer hip fractures than the placebo group, and 32% fewer fractures in areas outside the hip and spine.[23]

These results are remarkable, especially when you consider that estrogen replacement therapy generally reduces a woman's fracture risk by 50%.

Combining Estrogen with Calcium and Vitamin D

If a woman is taking estrogen replacement therapy (ERT), can she also benefit by taking calcium supplements? A recent review of research on this question tells us that she definitely can. An analysis of 31 studies showed that a regimen of estrogen plus about 1,200 mg of calcium daily was more effective at protecting against bone loss than taking estrogen alone.[24] What about adding vitamin D into the mix? A recent study combined calcium and vitamin D supplements with low-dosage hormone replacement therapy (HRT). The study involved 128 women over age 65 with low bone mass. They received either placebo or a dose of HRT equivalent to 0.3 mg per day of conjugated equine estrogen plus 2.5 mg per day of medroxyprogesterone. This dosage of estrogen was a little less than half the amount of estrogen that is generally found to be effective for protecting bone.[25] All 128 women also received calcium and vitamin D supplements, enough to bring their total calcium consumption from all sources up to 1,000 mg daily.

After 3½ years, the women who had received HRT plus the calcium and vitamin D supplements showed significant increases in bone density in the spine, total body, and forearm. According to researchers, one possible explanation is that calcium and vitamin D deficiencies are so common among postmenopausal women that the effectiveness of HRT can be greatly improved just by correcting this deficiency.

So even if you take estrogen, you should take these supplements as well. You may also be able to get by with a lower dose of estrogen, one that should present less risk of breast cancer.

What About Osteoporosis Caused by Medications?

One of the most serious side effects of long-term use of corticosteroid drugs is accelerated osteoporosis. According to one preliminary study, taking extra calcium (1 g daily) might help reduce the risk of corticosteroid-induced osteoporosis.[26] In another study, taking both calcium (1 g daily) and vitamin D (500 IU daily) while taking a corticosteroid protected against bone loss.[27] In addition, anti-seizure medications such as Dilantin and phenobarbitol may lower the levels of calcium and/or vitamin D in the body and you may need to take extra amounts of these nutrients to protect your bone health.[28,29] However, because excessive amounts of vitamin D may have toxic effects in the body, supplementation with vitamin D requires prudence.[30] (See the safety precautions in Interactions with Medications later in this chapter.)

Calcium and Vitamin D Supplements: What Kind and How Much?

Now that you've seen the evidence on calcium and vitamin D, you might want to know more about these supplements and how to take them.

Calcium Dosage

See table 2 for a list of recommendations of calcium intakes for various age groups. Establishing nutritional requirements isn't an exact science, and these numbers are specifically designed for *optimal calcium intake:* to maximize the building of peak bone mass in childhood and young adulthood, and to minimize bone loss in adulthood.

Table 2: Recommended Calcium Intakes

Age (years)	Calcium (mg/day)
Birth–6 months	210
6 months–1 year	270
1–3	500
4–8	800
9–18	1,300
19–50	1,000
51 and older	1,200
Pregnant or nursing women	1,000 (1,300 if age 18 or younger)

Are All Calcium Supplements the Same?

Calcium supplements come in several different forms, each with its own advantages and drawbacks: naturally derived calcium (dolomite, bonemeal, oyster shell); refined calcium carbonate; and chelated calcium (calcium citrate, calcium citrate malate, calcium gluconate, calcium lactate, and others).

Naturally Derived Calcium

Naturally derived calcium supplements come from bone, shells, or the earth. Also called "unrefined calcium carbonate," this type of supplement includes calcium from dolomite, bone meal, hydroxyapatite, and oyster shell. Aside from the appeal of a natural product, these supplements have two big advantages: they're inexpensive, and they're easier to swallow than other, bulkier forms. You can get as much as 500 to 600 mg in one rather small tablet.

But naturally derived calcium has a couple of drawbacks. It may be harder to absorb, and some natural sources of calcium may also contain significant amounts of lead. Lead is a toxic mineral that can cause damage to the nervous system, the kidneys, and the red blood cells, especially in children. Lead accumulates in the body, so even small amounts can build up to toxic levels over time.

A study published in 1993 reported the lead content of 70 different brands of calcium supplements.[31] Twenty-five percent of the products tested had lead levels *higher* than the FDA's "tolerable" intake for children ages 6 and under. Another 20% of the calcium supplements did not significantly exceed tolerable lead levels, but they did have more lead than is good for you (more than is allowable in milk, for example). The sources highest in lead were bonemeal, dolomite, and oyster shell—all the leading sources of unrefined calcium carbonate.

The popular supplement hydroxyapatite falls into this category, too, because it's made from bonemeal. Some manufacturers of this product claim that their source is lead-free, but this claim is hard to verify when you're standing in the aisle at your pharmacy. Calcium supplements rarely list the lead content of their source, but they should. The lead concentration should always be less than 2 parts per million.

Calcium Carbonate

Refined calcium carbonate is the least expensive form of calcium, because it's nothing but refined limestone, chemically identical to chalk. Like its earthier cousins, refined calcium carbonate is easier to swallow than chelated supplements, in which calcium is chemically bound to an organic acid. These chelated molecules are bulky compared to the calcium carbonate molecule. This means that a pill containing 500 mg of calcium carbonate, refined or unrefined, is much smaller than a 500 mg calcium citrate supplement. Furthermore, the refining process seems to eliminate most of the lead. In the study mentioned previously, refined calcium carbonate was found to contain up to the "tolerable" limit of about 1 mcg per 800 mg.

Calcium carbonate, for all its advantages, isn't perfect. It often causes constipation (usually mild), and because it is an antacid, using it over the long run may cause the stomach to respond by producing more acid, leading to "rebound hyperacidity" and stomach irritation.

A major issue with calcium carbonate is how well it dissolves in the digestive tract. If a calcium pill doesn't dissolve there, it will pass right through you, doing you no good at all. A study of 27 brands of calcium carbonate found that the extent of dissolving varied from 33% to 75%. If a tablet is only 33% dissolved, it means that two-thirds of the calcium will pass through your body without helping you.[32] However, one of the most common ways to take refined calcium carbonate is in a chewable over-the-counter antacid tablet. Obviously, this form is pretty effectively dissolved before it reaches your intestines.

Another issue is how well your body absorbs the calcium from a given supplement. Calcium carbonate requires acid in order to dissolve at all (the test-tube research mentioned previously used an acidic solution), and some people may not have enough acid in their stomach. This is especially true of the elderly, as well as those taking medications such as Zantac, Pepcid, and Prilosec that dramatically decrease acid secretion. Taking calcium carbonate supplements with meals helps

A study of 27 brands of calcium carbonate found that the extent of dissolving varied from 33% to 75%. If a tablet is only 33% dissolved, it means that two-thirds of the calcium will pass through your body without helping you.

to some extent, because that is when your stomach acid levels are highest.

The research mentioned previously also indicates that calcium carbonate has another disadvantage. It may be less effective against bone loss than the *chelated* forms of calcium supplements that are described next.

Chelated Calcium

Chelated calcium is calcium bound to an organic acid. Several different forms of calcium come under this category, including citrate, citrate malate, lactate, gluconate, aspartate, and orotate.

Although chelated calcium is bulkier than calcium carbonate, it dissolves easily and (at least in the calcium citrate form) may be easier to absorb.[33] As we've mentioned, one study compared the effects of calcium carbonate and calcium citrate malate in postmenopausal women.[34] The calcium citrate malate proved more effective in slowing bone loss. While the calcium carbonate slowed bone loss only in the wrists, the chelated form of calcium gave significant protection to the spine as well. These results were recently presented at a meeting of the American Society for Bone and Mineral Research. In this study of women in early menopause, 800 mg daily of calcium citrate stabilized bone mineral density in the spine and other parts of the skeleton.[35] Another study on adolescents found that calcium citrate malate was absorbed significantly better than calcium carbonate. Overall, the increase in the level of calcium ab-

Although chelated calcium is bulkier than calcium carbonate, it dissolves easily and (at least in the calcium citrate form) may be easier to absorb.

How Much Calcium Should You Take at Once?

Calcium absorption studies have found that we can absorb only about 500 mg of calcium from a supplement at any given time. If you're taking more than 500 mg daily, it's best to split it up into two or more doses, preferably at mealtimes.

sorbed was 36% for the chelated form compared to only a 26% increase in absorption for the calcium carbonate form.[36] Depending on your source, though, chelated calcium supplements may be expensive enough to justify taking higher amounts of calcium carbonate. One increasingly common source of calcium citrate malate is also fairly inexpensive: calcium-fortified orange juice.

Vitamin D Dosage

Unlike calcium, which is measured by weight, vitamin D is measured in international units (IU). The recommended daily intake of vitamin D is between 200 and 400 IU (see table 3). You need only a little exposure to sunlight each day to get this amount—about 15 minutes without sunscreen. Vitamin D-fortified milk has 100 IU per cup. The major food source of vitamin D, cod liver oil, is unpopular, so most people deficient in vitamin D prefer to take a supplement.

But the medical community is currently debating whether the recommended amount is enough. A recent editorial in the *New England Journal of Medicine* states, "On the basis of what we know about vitamin D, sick adults, older adults, and perhaps all adults probably need 800 to 1,000 IU daily, substantially higher than the newly established levels of adequate intake."[37] Still, you should be careful not to take too much vitamin D.

Unlike calcium, various vitamin D supplements are all thought to work about the same, with similar advantages

Table 3. Recommended Vitamin D Intakes

Age (years)	Vitamin D (IU/day)
Birth–50	200
51–70	400
71 and older	600
Pregnant or nursing women	200

and disadvantages. The main problem with vitamin D is that it is toxic at excessive dosages, and it can accumulate in your body over time. See Safety Issues later in this chapter for more information.

Safety Issues

In general, calcium is considered safe to take at dosages up to 2,000 mg daily.[38] But people with certain illnesses, including cancer, hyperparathyroidism, or sarcoidosis, shouldn't take calcium supplements except under a doctor's supervision.

People with a history of kidney stones are often cautioned not to take supplemental calcium, because kidney stones are commonly made of calcium oxalate crystals. One recent study found that calcium supplements might indeed increase kidney stone risk (especially if the supplements are not taken with meals), but the same is not necessarily true for increasing your intake of calcium from food sources.[39] In fact, some studies show that the risk for kidney stones actually goes *down* when dietary calcium is increased.[40] Still, if you have a history of kidney stones, consult your physician before taking extra calcium.

Vitamin D becomes toxic at high dosages, leading to serious problems involving excess calcium in the blood and calcium deposits in internal organs. While toxicity is usually not seen below a dose of 2,400 IU daily, chronic intake of over 1,200 IU daily might eventually lead to problems. To be on the safe side, you should consult a doctor if you want to take more than 800 IU daily.

Interactions with Other Nutrients

Calcium supplements (or taking calcium-containing antacids) may reduce the absorption of a number of minerals, including zinc, chromium, and iron.[41–48] Though a number of studies have conflicting results, in some cases it appears that calcium-containing antacids may also reduce the absorption of manganese. However, researchers are not sure of the health significance of this finding.[49,50]

In general, to avoid potential problems with the absorption of zinc, chromium, iron, or manganese supplements, consider taking them 2 to 3 hours apart from calcium supplements or calcium-containing antacids and meals.

A chemical found in soy called phytic acid can also interfere with the absorption of calcium, so you should wait at least 2 hours after eating soy products before taking calcium.

The bottom line: When you are taking calcium, it is especially important to make sure you're getting enough of these nutrients, either in your diet or through a supplement.

Interactions with Medications

If you are taking certain medications, it may be especially important to get enough calcium and vitamin D. However, sometimes you have to be careful, as these supplements can also interfere with the absorption or action of various medications.

Anticonvulsant Medications

Calcium supplementation may be prudent if you are taking anticonvulsant drugs like carbamazepine because they may impair calcium absorption and interfere with bone formation and maintenance. However, calcium carbonate might interfere with the absorption of phenytoin and perhaps other anticonvulsants.[51–54] For this reason, if you are taking calcium supplements and anticonvulsant drugs, take them several hours apart if possible, and make sure that your health care provider is monitoring the blood levels of your medication and any seizure activity very closely.

Phenytoin and other anticonvulsant drugs like phenobarbital, primidone, and carbamazepine (and possibly valproic acid), may also interfere with vitamin D activity. This may lead to an impairment in calcium use by the body and a potential increase in the risk of osteoporosis and related bone disorders.[55–59] Interestingly, in many cases, adequate sun exposure may compensate for any loss of vitamin D activity that may be caused by anticonvulsant medicines. If you're concerned that you're not getting enough vitamin D this way, speak with your health care provider about taking vitamin D supplements.

Corticosteroid Medications

Corticosteroids taken for conditions like asthma cause osteoporosis by decreasing intestinal absorption of calcium. Studies have shown that taking calcium and vitamin D supplements may help prevent the loss of bone density associated with long-term corticosteroid therapy.[60,61] For this reason, if you are currently on long-term corticosteroid therapy (including the use of inhaled corticosteroids), calcium and vitamin D supplementation may help prevent bone mineral density loss, as well as fractures in the spine.

Antibiotics

Taking calcium supplements may interfere with the effectiveness of antibiotics in the tetracycline family.[62] In addition, dairy products or antacids containing calcium may decrease the absorption of some fluoroquinolone anti-biotics like norfloxacin or ciprofloxacin.[63,64] Because of this, calcium supplements and milk should be taken as far apart as possible from fluoroquinolone antibiotics. Calcium-containing antacids should be taken at least 6 hours before or 2 hours after quinolone antibiotics.

Cardiac Medications

Calcium supplements appear to interfere with the absorption of the drug atenolol and perhaps other drugs in the same beta-blocker family.[65]

There is also evidence that calcium may interfere with some of the effects of calcium channel blockers (like Verapamil), particularly their ability to reduce blood pressure.[66] While most of the research relates to calcium given intravenously, it is possible that calcium taken orally (especially when combined with vitamin D) might produce a similar effect.[67–71] Interestingly, physicians sometimes deliberately recommend calcium supplementation during treatment with calcium channel blockers to minimize unwanted blood pressure reduction. It is *extremely important* that you consult your physician before taking calcium or vitamin D supplements if you are currently taking calcium channel blockers. You will need to be closely monitored for any possible reduction in the effectiveness of your treatment.

Thiazide diuretics are a type of cardiac medication that decreases the amount of calcium excreted in the urine. Because of this, when they are combined with supplemental calcium, blood levels of calcium may become dangerously high. This is especially the case if you are also taking vitamin D supplements or have a medical condition known as hyperparathyroidism.[72–75] Make sure that your health care provider is aware that you are taking calcium or vitamin D supplements with thiazide diuretics.

Finally, there is weak evidence that the heart medicine digoxin may cause calcium depletion. However, researchers are not sure of the health significance of this finding[76] or whether calcium supplementation would be helpful if you are taking digoxin. In general, though, it seems reasonable to make sure that you are getting adequate amounts of calcium either through diet or supplements.

Medicines for Gastrointestinal Distress

Concerns have been raised that the aluminum in aluminum-containing antacids may present a health risk. In addition, there is evidence that calcium citrate and other citrates may increase the absorption of aluminum from antacids as well as from dietary sources, thus increasing the risk.[77,78] Given these concerns and to help minimize potential toxicity, consider avoiding aluminum-containing antacids if you are taking calcium citrate.

At the very least, take calcium citrate supplements apart from aluminum-containing antacids and meals.

Some research suggests that cimetidine, a medicine used to decrease the production of acid in the stomach, may interfere with vitamin D metabolism.[79,80,81] If you are taking cimetidine on a long term basis, vitamin D supplementation at nutritional levels may be needed.

Anticoagulants

High dose or long-term use of the anti-clotting medicine heparin may interfere with the conversion of dietary vitamin D to its active form in the body, possibly causing bone mineral loss that may lead to osteoporosis. Some studies of pregnant women found heparin therapy to be associated with fractured and collapsed vertebra.[82,83,84] Calcium and vitamin D supplementation may help prevent heparin-induced osteoporosis. If you are taking long term heparin therapy, consider having your bone density monitored routinely.

Medicines for Tuberculosis

Some research suggests that the antituberculosis drug isoniazid (either alone or in combination with the drug rifampin) may interfere with the activity of vitamin D, leading to decreased blood levels of calcium and phosphate.[85,86] Because of this, if you are taking isoniazid alone or in combination with rifampin, it may be necessary for you to have your calcium and vitamin D levels monitored. As always, speak with your health care provider about what's best for you.

Ipriflavone and Phytoestrogens

Estrogen plays an instrumental role in protecting women's bones. After menopause, a woman's natural levels of estrogen fall, and her bone mass may decline sharply as a result. Estrogen replacement therapy (ERT) and hormone replacement therapy (HRT) are two ways to maintain the body's levels of estrogen after menopause. In addition to protecting bone, estrogen might have other helpful effects, such as reducing the risk for heart disease.

But many women prefer not to take estrogen. Because it may increase a woman's risk for breast cancer, estrogen is not recommended for cancer survivors or women at high risk. There are also other health conditions that can rule out estrogen replacement therapy. (See chapter 9 for a more detailed discussion of estrogen and hormone replacement therapy.)

In the following sections we also examine ipriflavone, an alternative treatment that appears to possess the osteoporosis-fighting power of estrogen without its drawbacks.

Ipriflavone is a dietary supplement produced in the laboratory from soy isoflavones.

Phytoestrogens

A *phytoestrogen* is a plant-based chemical compound that has an effect in the human body similar to that of a very weak estrogen. Over 300 different plant species have been identified as containing phytoestrogens, one of these being the soybean. In your body, phytoestrogens bind to *estrogen receptor sites,* which are where estrogen would normally attach itself to the cells it affects. There are estrogen receptor sites in the uterus, breasts, nervous system, and brain. Unlike estrogen, the phytoestrogens' ability to bind to these receptor sites is weak. As a result, the plant-based "estrogens" have a less potent effect

Ipriflavone is a dietary supplement produced in the laboratory from soy isoflavones.

in the body. For example, the phytoestrogens found in soybeans have ⅟₁₀₀ to ⅟₁,₀₀₀ the activity of estradiol, the most powerful naturally occurring estrogen.

Because of this difference, phytoestrogens may be able to either increase or decrease the activity of estrogen in various sites of the body. Where estrogen levels are higher than normal, phytoestrogens may bind with some of the estrogen receptor sites and thus block some of the body's own estrogen. The result is a lower estrogen effect. But where the body's levels of estrogen are low, the phytoestrogens may weakly increase the overall effect of estrogen. A type of phytoestrogen found in soybeans is called an *isoflavone.*

Isoflavones

In the last decade, phytoestrogens have attracted attention because of their possible role in inhibiting certain forms of cancer and reducing the risk for coronary heart disease.[1,2] They have also been investigated as possible treatments for osteoporosis.

Researchers have found that postmenopausal Asian women had lower rates of hip fracture than white women in America. Yet they were less likely to use estrogen replacement therapy, and their diets included less calcium. Some scientific evidence suggests an interesting explanation for why Asian women, like those in Japan, experience a lower rate of hip fractures: their relatives take such good care of them that they are simply less likely to suffer a fall. Beyond the positive impact of family interactions, researchers have also investigated links between the Japanese diet and bone loss.[3] The evidence suggests that soy isoflavones might be part of the answer. Soybeans are an important staple in the Japanese diet. Tofu, fermented soybean products such as miso and tempeh, and green soybeans are some of the many forms in which soybeans appear in Japan's cuisine. As a result,

> **In the last decade, phytoestrogens have attracted attention because of their possible role in inhibiting certain forms of cancer and reducing the risk for coronary heart disease.[1,2] They have also been investigated as possible treatments for osteoporosis.**

Table 4. Isoflavone Content of Soy Foods[5]

Source	Serving Size	Isoflavones Per Serving (mg)
Roasted soybeans	½ cup	167
Soy flour	¼ cup	44
Textured soy protein	¼ cup	28
Soymilk	1 cup	20
Tempeh, uncooked	4 oz	60
Tofu, uncooked	4 oz	38
Soy protein powder	1 oz	57
Green soybeans, uncooked	½ cup	70

Japanese women may consume 150 to 200 mg of soy isoflavones in their diet every day.[4] Although other Asian countries consume less soy than Japan, their inhabitants still eat much more than the typical North American, who gets less than 5 mg of soy isoflavones daily (see table 4).

Two of the most common and well-researched soy isoflavones are *genistein* and *daidzein*. Animal research has shown that at low doses, genistein is as effective as estrogen in maintaining bone density in rats whose ovaries have been removed.[6] While we can't assume that what's good for a rat will work equally well for a human, there is at least a good reason to investigate whether isoflavones protect people's bones, too.

One published study looked at the effects of isoflavonoid-rich soy protein on human bone density.[7] In this study, 66 postmenopausal women took either 56 mg or 90 mg of soy isoflavones for 6 months. A control group took a milk protein formula which contained no soy isoflavones. After 6 months, the group that took the higher dosage of soy isoflavones had significant gains in bone density in the spine compared to the group that received no isoflavones. The group taking the smaller dosage of soy isoflavones had only an insignificant gain.

Three longer studies on soy isoflavones and bone density are currently underway in the United States. When they're published, we'll have better information on the effects of natural soy isoflavones on bone density. The evidence for soy isoflavones is promising, but further studies are needed to give more definitive answers as to what impact soy isoflavones have on bone, heart, and breast health.

Safety Issues

A food that has been around for centuries, soy is generally considered to be safe. (This is not true, however, for raw soybeans, which contain a toxin that is neutralized by cooking and processing.)

But the jury is still out when it comes to the safety of phytoestrogens for women who have had breast cancer. While many studies suggest that eating soy might lower one's risk for breast cancer,[8,9,10] there is also some evidence that it may have the opposite effect, actually increasing the risk.[11] Until there is better, more conclusive evidence one way or the other, women with breast cancer or at high risk for it should approach soy isoflavones with caution. In general, eating soy foods is probably a safer approach than taking high-dosage isoflavone supplements. Remember that isoflavones in general act like very weak estrogens in the body. We suspect that natural isoflavones are most helpful in middle-range dosages. Small or large doses might not have as beneficial an effect, or might even be harmful.

Dosage

For naturally occurring isoflavones from food, the best dosage isn't known. We know that Japanese women eat up to 200 mg of soy isoflavones daily, but we don't know whether this is the ideal amount for maintaining strong bones.

Soy Isoflavones Are Good for You in Other Ways

Aside from protecting bone, soy isoflavones have been shown to lower cholesterol levels, ease "hot flashes" and other symptoms of menopause, and possibly help prevent cancer of the breast and prostate.[12] In one study, three groups of postmenopausal women following a low-fat, low-cholesterol diet also received a protein supplement containing a high dose of soy isoflavones, a low dose of soy isoflavones, or no isoflavones. Women receiving the isoflavone supplements had reductions in their cholesterol levels as well as an increase in their HDL or "good" cholesterol levels. The researchers concluded that soy protein may decrease the risk factors associated with heart disease in postmenopausal women.[13]

The suggested daily intake for food isoflavones is 50 mg daily. When pending research on the effects of isoflavones is completed, this recommendation may change.

Ipriflavone

Used today to prevent and treat osteoporosis in Japan, Hungary, and Italy, ipriflavone was specifically created to protect bone. The results of 150 studies have established it as an effective treatment for osteoporosis.

In 1969, a research project was initiated to manufacture a treatment that would possess the bone-stimulating effects of phytoestrogens without the estrogen activity. The purpose behind this search was to find a treatment that could prevent osteoporosis without incurring any of the risks involved in taking estrogen. The result was ipri-flavone, a supplement made from isoflavones found in soy-beans. The two major isoflavones in soybeans are called genistein and daidzein; both are very similar to ipriflavone in chemical structure (see figure 6).

Ipriflavone was specifically created to protect bone. The results of 150 studies have established it as an effective treatment for osteoporosis.

In the early 1970s, re-searchers tested ipriflavone on animals and found that it had an intriguing effect: It increased the total amount of calcium the ani-mals retained in their bones.[14]

After 7 successful years of experiments with animals, human research on ipriflavone began in 1981. Sixty studies later, with more than 2,700 human study participants, ipriflavone is now available in over 22 coun-tries. Although it is still not as well known in the United States, some drugstores and Web sites offer it as a nonprescription dietary supplement.

Ipriflavone and Your Bones

Like estrogen, ipriflavone seems to protect bone by in-hibiting the growth of osteoclasts, the cells that cause bone resorption. But, as its inventors intended, it doesn't seem to have any of estrogen's effects elsewhere in the body.[15,16] This means that it won't ease the hot flashes, vaginal dry-ness, or mood swings that often accompany menopause; then again, it won't make these symptoms worse. More im-portantly, ipriflavone appears to have *no* effect on breast tissue. This strongly suggests that, unlike estrogen, it shouldn't increase your risk for breast cancer. (See Safety Issues later in this chapter for more information.)

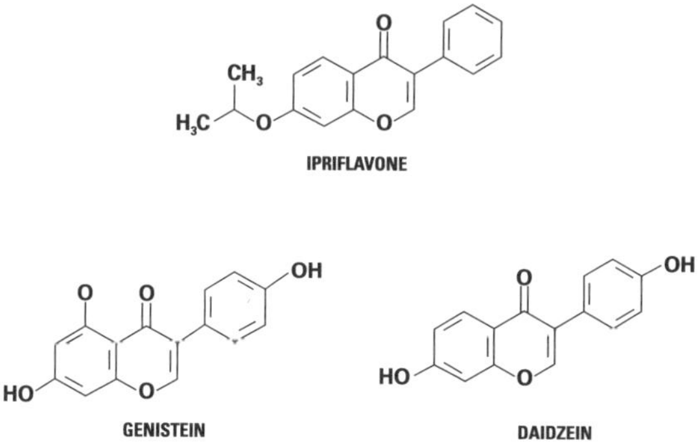

Figure 6. *Chemical structures of ipriflavone, daidzein, and genistein*

Ipriflavone also stimulates new bone formation. In cell cultures, it has been shown to help regulate the growth of osteoblasts (the cells that build new bone), increasing the amount of calcium put into the bone and also helping the body produce the proteins of the bone matrix.[17,18] (Bone is made primarily of calcium crystals bound in a *matrix* of collagen and other proteins and minerals. Ipriflavone enhances the production of these bone proteins, which are needed for a healthy matrix.[18,19])

Animal studies have found that ipriflavone increases bone density without altering the composition of bone or the structure of the calcium crystals. This suggests that ipriflavone helps strengthen bone density while maintaining the normal composition of bone.[19]

How Effective Is Ipriflavone?

Test-tube and animal studies suggest that ipriflavone may have a bone-protecting effect similar to estrogen's. But only properly designed trials on human beings can tell us whether it really works, and how well. Fortunately, ipriflavone has been extensively studied as a treatment for osteoporosis: 60 human studies have been conducted, about 20 of which used the optimum double-blind placebo-controlled design. The results of these studies indicate that ipriflavone effectively stops bone loss in the spine as well as other parts of the skeleton. Some results suggest that it even builds bone.

In one study, 60 postmenopausal women who had already been diagnosed with osteoporosis and had suffered at least one spinal fracture were divided into two groups. One group received 600 mg of ipriflavone in 3 daily doses of 200 mg, while the other group received placebo. In addition, both groups received 1,000 mg of calcium carbonate daily. After 6 months, the group that received ipriflavone and calcium had an increase in spinal bone density of 3.5%. The placebo and calcium group, however, lost bone density (-2.1%). Thus, ipriflavone had an overall effect of improving spinal bone density by 5.6%.[20]

Ipriflavone effectively stops bone loss in the spine as well as other parts of the skeleton.

You probably aren't surprised that the calcium alone didn't stop bone loss in the spine. We saw the same result in most of the studies on calcium described in chapter 4. This study showed that ipriflavone plus calcium could significantly rebuild spine tissue even after it was weakened by osteoporosis.

Other studies have found similar results. One included 40 women aged 47 to 65. All were menopausal, and all showed evidence of bone loss. Again, the women were split into two groups. As in the study mentioned previously, one group received placebo plus 1,000 mg of calcium, and the other received 600 mg ipriflavone plus the same dosage of calcium. (In this study, the researchers tried a

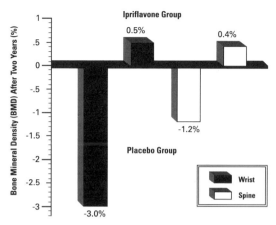

Figure 7. *Ipriflavone vs. placebo
in a two-year bone mass study*[23]

slightly different treatment regimen with the ipriflavone:
they provided it in two daily doses of 300 mg.) After 1 year,
the placebo group had lost an average of 2.2% of their
spinal density, while the ipriflavone group gained 1.2%, a
significant difference. In other words, ipriflavone protected a total of 3.4% of their spinal bone density.[21]

Two other large studies showed similar positive results. In one, 134 women aged 50 to 65 completed treatment with either ipriflavone or placebo (both groups also
received 1,000 mg of calcium carbonate).[22] At the comple-
tion of the two-year study, those who took ipriflavone had
gained, on average, a modest amount of bone in their
spine (0.4%), while the placebo group *lost* an average of
1.2%. In the other study, 453 postmenopausal women received either ipriflavone or placebo plus 1,000 mg of calcium carbonate. Women who received ipriflavone
maintained both spinal and forearm bone mass, while
women who received placebo had a significant decrease
(see figure 7).[23]

It's certainly good news that ipriflavone is effective at preventing postmenopausal bone loss, especially in the spine. However, because many women lose bone at a steep rate in the first 3 to 6 years after menopause, it's also worth knowing whether ipriflavone can help slow or stop bone loss at that time.

A smaller study looked specifically at 56 women who had begun menopause within the previous 5 years.[24] One group received 600 mg of ipriflavone daily and the other received placebo (both received 1,000 mg of supplemental calcium). After 2 years, those who took placebo lost 4.9% of their spinal bone mass, a significant loss. But the women who took ipriflavone had *no* significant changes in their spinal bone.

In addition, another small study of 91 postmenopausal women, including women in their early postmenopausal years, found that after 6 months women taking ipriflavone had an increase in their spinal bone mineral density while those in the placebo group had a decrease.[25]

Ipriflavone and Antiestrogen Medications

Certain medications can increase your risk for osteoporosis. *Gonadotropin-releasing hormone agonists* (GnRH agonists) are a type of medication used to treat uterine fibroids and endometriosis. These drugs work by stopping your body from producing estrogen. Unfortunately, this means that your bones lose the estrogen's protective effects, and you may lose bone mass. Bone loss may continue for up to 6 months after treatment with these medications.

Because it only mimics estrogen's bone-protecting effects, and doesn't act like estrogen in any other part of the body, ipriflavone may be able to help women who must take gonadotropin-releasing hormone agonists. And there is evidence suggesting that it does help substantially, without interfering with the medication.

In a double-blind placebo-controlled study, 100 pre-menopausal women with uterine fibroids were given a common GnRH agonist, a medication called Lupron.[26] Lupron was given by injection once every 30 days for 6 months. In addition, half of the women received 600 mg of ipriflavone each day and the other half received placebo (both groups also received 500 mg of calcium daily).

After 6 months, the women who took the placebo and calcium had lost almost 6% of their total bone mass, including 4% in the spine. This is a serious loss, comparable to the amount a woman might lose in a year just after menopause. And the women's bone mass didn't improve appreciably in the next 12 months, even when they were no longer receiving Lupron.

But the women taking ipriflavone lost no bone mass. Yet Lupron was just as effective in these women as in the placebo group, suggesting that the ipriflavone didn't interfere with the desired estrogen-suppressing effects of Lupron.

How Does Ipriflavone Compare to Other Treatments for Osteoporosis?

In the United States, the two most commonly used medications for treating osteoporosis are estrogen replacement therapy (ERT) and a drug called alendronate sodium (Fosamax). (As you may recall from earlier discussions, when ERT is combined with a progestin—a chemical cousin of the sex hormone progesterone—the combination is called "hormone replacement therapy," or HRT.)

Studies on hormone replacement therapy show increases of spinal bone density in the range of 4 to 5% in the first 2 years. Results for alendronate (using a typical dosage of 5 mg daily) are similar, with gains in the range of 3.5 to 5.5% for the first 2 to 3 years of treatment.[27,28] Since the control groups in these studies typically lost spinal bone mass (about 2%), the actual benefit of both alendronate and HRT should be measured by the total bone saved and bone gained. The total benefit of both Fosamax and HRT includes not only this added bone mass, but also the bone *loss* the medications prevented.

How does ipriflavone compare to these treatments? Unfortunately, we can't say for certain. The only way to accurately compare the effectiveness of two treatments is to set up a double-blind placebo-controlled study on both treatments. At the present, all we have is the evidence of separate studies. From a scientific point of view, you can't exactly compare the results of separate studies, because the participants involved may be different in various important ways. Still, you can get a ballpark estimate of comparative effectiveness this way.

In the ipriflavone studies that have been performed, the overall benefit seen ranged from 0.5% to over 7% (probably due to differences in the groups of women enrolled in each study).[29] This puts ipriflavone in the same general range of effectiveness as conventional treatments.

Does Ipriflavone Prevent Fractures?

It's all very well to know that ipriflavone stops bone loss and builds bone in women with osteoporosis, but shouldn't that mean it also prevents or reduces fractures? It should, based on what we know already, but it's always nice to know the bottom-line result of a treatment. Estrogen and alendronate, for example, have been found to decrease fracture rates by about 30 to 50%. (In other words, they cut an individual's risk by a third to a half.)

Two studies thus far have examined ipriflavone's effect on fracture rates. These studies both showed that ipriflavone significantly reduced the risk of fracture—but they were small studies, and need to be repeated on a larger scale before the results are conclusive.[30,31] Both studies were double-blind placebo-controlled trials with women who already had osteoporosis and showed signs of at least one fracture. None of the women had received treatment for their bone loss before the study. In one of these studies, 49 women with osteoporosis (age 65–79) took either 600 mg of ipriflavone daily or a placebo pill.[30] As we have seen in many of the studies mentioned previously, all of the participants took 1,000 mg calcium daily as well. After 2 years, an analysis of these women's fracture rates showed impressive results: the fracture rate was reduced by 50% in the ipriflavone group compared to the placebo group. In addition, the bone density in the wrists of women taking ipriflavone had increased by 7%. Of interest as well is that researchers also noted a reduction in pain during treatment with ipriflavone.[31] They found that pain was lessened and that ipriflavone's pain-relieving action continued throughout the treatment period. In addition, not only was the amount of drugs that the women required to relieve pain reduced, but their mobility improved also. Other clinical trials support these findings of pain reduction with ipriflavone as well.[32–35]

Though these results are promising, only larger studies can tell us for certain whether ipriflavone reduces the risk of fracture as effectively as estrogen or alendronate.

More evidence will be forthcoming from a large clinical study that began in Europe in 1997. The Ipriflavone Multicenter European Fracture Study will examine the effects of ipriflavone on women's fracture rates due to osteoporosis. The study is due to be completed in 2001.

Can Ipriflavone Help You Cut Your Dosage of Estrogen?

Because of the risks of estrogen therapy, many women would like to use as low a dose as possible. As with calcium and vitamin D, there is some evidence that ipriflavone can enhance the osteoporosis-fighting effects of estrogen.

For example, one study examined low dosages of estrogen in combination with ipriflavone.[36] The women in this study had recently entered menopause (within 6 months to 2 years), and had not received any supplemental estrogen for 6 months before the study. They also had at least two risk factors for osteoporosis (see chapter 2 for information on risk factors), as well as evidence of current bone loss. These 109 women were randomly divided into four groups and received one of the following:

1. 0.15 mg of a conjugated estrogen (Premarin) plus placebo
2. 0.30 mg of a conjugated estrogen (Premarin) plus placebo
3. 0.15 mg of a conjugated estrogen (Premarin) plus 600 mg of ipriflavone (200 mg three times daily)
4. 0.30 mg of a conjugated estrogen (Premarin) plus 600 mg of ipriflavone (200 mg three times daily)

In addition, all of the women were given 1,000 mg calcium daily and a progestin for a 15-day period every 3 months.

This study's results showed that the combination of 600 mg ipriflavone and 0.3 mg conjugated estrogens worked much better than the same low (0.3 mg) dosage of estrogen alone. The women taking both ipriflavone and estrogen had relief from hot flashes and other menopausal symptoms, and at the end of the 12-month study their wrist bone density had increased by 5.6%—significantly better results than were seen for the women taking estrogen (0.3 mg) without ipriflavone. The women who took estrogen alone *lost* bone density, though not enough for the results to be significant.

Another study compared ipriflavone and estrogen separately against a combined therapy using both.[37] This study looked at women whose ovaries had been removed (a high risk group for osteoporosis, since their bone mass can decrease by as much as 8 to 10% *each year* in the first few years after the surgery). These 116 women were divided into four groups, each of which received one of the following:

1. placebo
2. 0.625 mg estrogen daily
3. 600 mg ipriflavone daily
4. 0.625 mg estrogen plus 600 mg ipriflavone daily

Taken separately, the estrogen and ipriflavone had similar results: Neither estrogen nor ipriflavone was able to prevent bone loss. But when taken together, ipriflavone plus estrogen stopped bone loss. Women who took both finished the 48-week study without any significant loss in bone mineral density. These results suggest that for women who are at serious risk for bone loss, or who cannot tolerate dosages of estrogen higher than 0.625 mg, combining estrogen with ipriflavone might be helpful.

Despite these promising findings, we do need to add one note of caution: At least one animal study suggests that when ipriflavone is taken with estrogen, it might enhance estrogen's effect on the uterine lining.[38] This might mean that ipriflavone would enhance the risk of endometrial cancer, and perhaps other health risks associated with estrogen replacement therapy. Unfortunately, very little research has been conducted that would shed light on this important question. Until more evidence is available, we can't recommend that you combine ipriflavone with estrogen replacement therapy except under the close supervision of a qualified health care professional.

Dosage

The proper dosage of ipriflavone has been well established through numerous studies: 600 mg daily, taken in

Do Isoflavones in Food Work As Well As Ipriflavone?

Much less research has been done on the bone-protecting effects of naturally occurring isoflavones in soybeans and other foods. The fact that ipriflavone is chemically very similar to the soy isoflavones daidzein and genistein suggests that there might be similar effects.

Not enough studies have been done, however, to prove that the two are equivalent in their bone-saving properties.

Soy isoflavones appear to be good for you in general, and it probably wouldn't hurt to eat more of them (refer to table 4).

two or three separate doses. (But a lower dosage is necessary for people with kidney disease. Consult your physician for more information.)

Safety Issues

The safety of ipriflavone has been studied extensively. Over 2,700 people have been treated with ipriflavone in 60 studies that generally lasted at least 1 year. In general, ipriflavone seems to be extremely safe. It produced fewer side effects than placebo. An average of 14.5% of study participants taking ipriflavone complained of side effects (mostly mild gastrointestinal complaints), compared with 16% of those taking placebo. (Placebo treatments, the inactive pills researchers give to study participants who aren't getting the real treatment, have a well-known power to make people feel better. They also do just the opposite. For some people, simply taking a pill is enough to give them a stomachache. However, in this case, it's also possible that the study participants were feeling the effects of the 1,000 mg calcium carbonate that accompanied the treatment.)

Of the 2,769 study participants who have taken ipriflavone in studies, 6% were taken off the medication because of side effects. In every case, the side effects disappeared when the medication and calcium were stopped.[39]

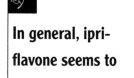

When taken alone, ipriflavone appears to have no effect on the uterus, brain, breast, or vaginal tissue of postmenopausal women, or the thyroid gland or uterus of experimental animals.[40] While the risk of developing breast cancer or other forms of cancer that are sensitive to estrogen's actions in the body does not seem likely from current research,[41–44] we believe that caution is warranted, especially in women who have already had an occurrence of breast cancer or a cancer of their reproductive organs, or in women who are being treated with combinations of hormones and ipriflavone.

In general, ipriflavone seems to be extremely safe.

So what's the bottom line here? In the absence of long-term safety studies (such as the ones that have been done on estrogen), it isn't possible to say for certain that ipriflavone does *not* increase the risk of breast cancer. Women who have had breast cancer or who are currently using ERT or HRT should definitely consult a qualified health care practitioner before taking ipriflavone.

Because ipriflavone is eliminated by the kidneys, there is some concern that the recommended dosage of 600 mg daily might not be safe for those with kidney disease. A lower dosage (200 to 400 mg daily) is recommended for people whose kidneys are compromised in any way. Anyone with kidney disease or a history of kidney problems should take ipriflavone only under a doctor's supervision.

Other Important Nutrients for Your Bones

I n chapter 4 we showed you how calcium and vitamin D work to protect and build bone. Other vitamins and minerals are involved in the development of bone as well, including vitamin K, magnesium, vitamin B_6, and several trace minerals. Many natural health practitioners recommend a balanced intake of all of these nutrients as part of an approach to preventing osteoporosis. This is a common-sense way to take care of your general health as well as your bone health. Table 6 lists common sources of many of these vitamins and minerals. Table 5 provides both therapeutic dose recommendations for those with osteoporosis and general dietary recommended doses of these vitamins and minerals for men and women age 51 and over.

Vitamin K

Vitamin K is most important for its role in helping blood to clot, but it also plays a significant role in bone forma-

Table 5. Dietary and Therapeutic Dosage Recommendations for Selected Nutrients

Nutrient	General Dietary Recommended Level, Age 51 and Over		Therapeutic Dosage for Osteoporosis
	Male	Female	
Magnesium	420 mg	320 mg	300–600 mg
Vitamin K	80 mcg	65 mcg	150–500 mcg
Vitamin B$_6$°	2.0 mg	1.6 mg	10–300 mg
Manganese	2–5 mg	2–5 mg	3–6 mg
Boron	1.5–3 mg	1.5–3 mg	3 mg
Zinc°°	15 mg	12mg	12–15 mg
Copper	1.5–3 mg	1.5–3 mg	1–3 mg
Silicon°°°	20 mg	40 mg	Not known

Note: General Dietary Recommended Level refers to the U.S. Recommended Dietary Allowances or recognized "safe and adequate" levels. Therapeutic dosage refers to the range of intake suggested by the literature for the treatment of specific illnesses.

° We recommend not to exceed 50 mg of vitamin B$_6$ because of potential health issues

°° Doses exceeding 100 mg of zinc can be toxic

°°° We recommend not to exceed 50 mg of silicon

tion. A higher vitamin K intake appears to help prevent hip fractures.[1] A major protein found in our bones, *osteocalcin*, is thought to play an important role in the mineralization of bone. Vitamin K appears to be essential in converting osteocalcin to its active form in the bone.[2] There are three major forms of vitamin K. *Phylloquinone*

(K_1) is the natural form found in plants and the major form found in human bone; vitamin K_2 (menaquinone) is produced from bacteria in the gut; and vitamin K_3 (menadione) is a synthetic form. Severe vitamin K deficiency is rare. Recent evidence suggests that a higher intake of vitamin K than was previously thought necessary may help prevent osteoporosis.

Food Sources

The major dietary source of vitamin K is the plant form, K_1 (phylloquinone). Chlorophyll, the green substance found in plants, is an excellent source of vitamin K_1. As you'd expect, green leafy vegetables such as kale, parsley, spinach, broccoli, brussels sprouts, and lettuce are among the richest sources of vitamin K.

What Is the Scientific Evidence for Vitamin K and Osteoporosis?

A study 15 years ago found that people with low circulating phylloquinone (K_1) levels had an increased risk of osteoporotic hip fractures.[3] In addition, other studies have linked low blood levels of vitamin K with osteoporosis and hip fracture.[4–7] Vitamin K supplementation, on the other hand, has been associated with a reduction in the risk of hip fracture[8] as well as decreased calcium loss in the urine.[9–11] (A decrease in the loss of calcium through the urine is indirect evidence of a beneficial effect on bone.)

One study from the Netherlands found that vitamin K supplements of 1 mg daily improved the ability of osteocalcin (an important protein in bone) to bind to calcium crystals in postmenopausal women.[12] While the evidence from these studies suggests that vitamin K might play an important role in protecting bone, many were not well designed or large enough to conclusively prove anything.

A recent larger study has greatly strengthened the case for vitamin K. This well-designed ongoing observational study, the Nurses' Health Study, reported that postmenopausal women whose diets provided less than 109 mcg of vitamin K daily had significantly more hip fractures than women who took in a threshold level of 109 mcg.[13] The main dietary source of vitamin K was lettuce; women who ate lettuce (iceberg and romaine) at least once each day had a 45% lower risk of hip fracture than women who ate lettuce only once per week. The study authors noted that their method of determining vitamin K intake was only approximate, so the 109 mcg figure should not be taken too literally. However, this amount is about double the standard recommended allowance of 1 mcg per 2.2 pounds body weight. Based on this evidence, it seems that the RDA for vitamin K of 62 mcg per day might not be high enough to protect bone, and that a higher dosage than this might make a real difference.

Vitamin K is most important for its role in helping blood to clot, but it also plays a significant role in bone formation.

Another important finding from this study was that vitamin K did *not* seem to make a difference for women who were taking estrogen. This suggests that vitamin K might be most helpful for postmenopausal women who don't take supplemental estrogen.

Dosage

The RDA for vitamin K is 1 mcg per 2.2 pounds of body weight, or about 50 to 65 mcg daily for most women. As mentioned previously, a higher intake may be necessary to protect against osteoporosis.

Safety Issues

There are no known side effects associated with vitamin K, but individuals taking anticoagulant drugs (also known as "blood thinners") should not take additional vitamin K without consulting a physician, as the vitamin can undo the effect of those medications.

Magnesium

Magnesium is an essential mineral involved in hundreds of biochemical and cellular activities. Recently there's been growing interest in the role magnesium plays in bone metabolism.

The mineral component of bones consists mainly of calcium and phosphorus, and it also includes small amounts of magnesium, fluoride, sulfate, and other trace minerals. Some researchers have suggested that magnesium may be as important as calcium in the prevention and treatment of osteoporosis.

Magnesium plays several roles in the formation of bone. In animal studies, low dietary magnesium interfered with the normal formation of bone.[14] Magnesium is also thought to play an important role in the metabolism of vitamin D[15] and in the regulation of parathyroid hormone (PTH) which, in turn, stimulates bone cells (osteoclasts) to break down calcified bone in the cycle of bone remodeling.[16] (See chapter 1 for a description of this cycle.) And research also suggests that magnesium deficiency may result in decreased blood levels of the active form of vitamin D, as well as low levels of blood calcium and parathyroid hormone.[17] Finally, *alkaline phosphatase*, an enzyme involved in forming new bone, is activated by magnesium.[18]

While these observations don't prove anything on their own, they add to the evidence in favor of magnesium's importance in bone health.

Magnesium Deficiency

As you may have gathered from the previous discussion, we don't know for sure whether magnesium deficiency causes osteoporosis. But we do know that many of us don't get enough of this essential nutrient, and it seems logical to assume that a deficiency in magnesium isn't good for your bones. Mild deficiencies in magnesium seem to be extremely common in North America and Europe. One survey of "problem" nutrients in the United States found the lowest dietary magnesium intakes among females over the age of 11, teenage males, and in adults over 74 years of age.[19] Another review of the role of nutrition in osteoporosis reiterated the high likelihood that elderly individuals are magnesium-deficient.[20]

Why do so many of us get less magnesium than we should? One reason seems to be that modern processing strips magnesium from our food.[21] Whole grains are a good source of magnesium, but when they are refined, most of the magnesium is lost.

Certain medications and illnesses can also interfere with your ability to absorb and retain magnesium.[22] Chronic diarrhea, kidney disease, liver disease, diabetes, and pregnancy can also cause magnesium deficiency. It can also be caused by long-term use of certain medications, including some diuretics, oral contraceptives, and some heart medications. Other culprits of magnesium deficiency are excessive consumption of alcohol and aging.[23] As we age, our ability to absorb magnesium declines. At age 70, we absorb only 65% as much of the magnesium in our food as we do at age 30. Considering the prevalence of magnesium deficiency, it's probably worth making sure you get enough.

Factors Contributing to Magnesium Depletion

- Chronic use of digitalis, diuretics, or oral contraceptives
- High calcium intake
- Alcoholism
- Chronic diarrhea
- Diabetes
- Kidney disorders (renal tubular disorders)
- Pregnancy

Food Sources of Magnesium

Nuts, seeds, beans, tofu, green leafy vegetables, whole grains, and shrimp all contain elevated concentrations of magnesium. In comparison, meats and eggs contain relatively little magnesium.[24]

Sugars and fats have virtually no magnesium content. There is much less magnesium in refined grains (such as white flour and white rice) than in whole grains (such as whole wheat and brown rice). See Dosage for recommendations on using magnesium supplements.

What Is the Scientific Evidence for Magnesium?

There is some preliminary evidence suggesting possible links between magnesium and osteoporosis. A very small study involving 19 postmenopausal women with osteoporosis showed lower-than-normal magnesium levels in the hip and magnesium deficiencies in the blood.[25]

Another study examined 159 Caucasian women aged 23 to 75. The amount of magnesium in the diets of both premenopausal and postmenopausal women was found to significantly correlate with the bone mineral content of their forearms, suggesting that bone mass may indeed be affected by nutrients other than calcium.[26] A study of 194 postmenopausal women found that those who had osteoporosis had significantly lower dietary intake of calcium, phosphorus, and magnesium than the other women.[27] Larger, better-designed studies need to be done to fully determine whether magnesium supplementation can help prevent osteoporosis.

Dosage

Magnesium is available in several different forms, including citrate, malate, and aspartate. Studies indicate that magnesium is easily absorbed orally, especially when taken in a citrate form.[28] The RDA for magnesium is 320 to 420 mg daily. If your diet provides only 150 mg of magnesium on an average day, you'd need another 170 to 270 mg from a supplement to bring you up to the RDA. Because the RDA is only an approximation, and you personally may require more magnesium for optimum health, you may need to take as much as 500 mg of supplemental magnesium daily.

Magnesium is a safe, nontoxic supplement at the recommended dosage of 200 to 500 mg daily. When magnesium is taken over a long period of time, it needs to be balanced with other vitamins and minerals—especially calcium, phosphorus, and vitamin D. Though the best ratio of calcium to magnesium hasn't been determined, one study investigating the body's response to a combined calcium and magnesium supplement used a dosage of calcium that was twice as much as magnesium.[28] Consult with a knowledgeable health-care provider to determine your specific needs.

Safety Issues

As we mentioned previously, magnesium is safe to take at the recommended dosage of 200 to 500 mg daily. Citrate, malate, and aspartate forms of magnesium are recommended. Magnesium bound to inorganic salts such as carbonate, sulfate, oxide, or chloride often causes diarrhea at daily dosages higher than 200 mg.

> Though magnesium is a safe supplement, if you take it for a long period of time, you must be careful to balance your intake of magnesium with calcium, phosphorus, vitamin D, and other vitamins and minerals.

Though magnesium is a safe supplement, if you take it for a long period of time, you must be careful to balance your intake of magnesium with calcium, phosphorus, vitamin D, and other vitamins and minerals. Over the long term, excessive use of magnesium supplements has been known to cause abnormal bone mineralization, resulting in "softer" bones that are more susceptible to fractures.[29]

Those with severe kidney or heart disease should be cautious taking magnesium (or any other supplement) except on a doctor's recommendation. Pregnant women and those giving supplements to children should check with their health care provider before taking higher dosages of magnesium supplements.

Vitamin B$_6$ (Pyridoxine)

Vitamin B$_6$ is an important vitamin involved in many biological processes, including the transmission of nerve impulses, the formation of red blood cells and body proteins, and other functions. There is evidence that vitamin B$_6$ plays a role in bone formation and maintenance. Vitamin B$_6$ is a cofactor in the building of collagen, the protein that increases the strength of connective tissues, including bone tissue.

Vitamin B$_6$ Deficiency

The typical American diet provides less than the RDA for vitamin B$_6$.[30] Older people may be at even higher risk for B$_6$ deficiency; there is some evidence that they may not be able to absorb it well from food or supplements.[31]

Alcohol, food colorings, and various medications, including oral contraceptives, estrogen, progesterone, antibiotics in the tetracycline family, penicillamine, isoniazid, and hydralazine can all deplete your body's stores of vitamin B$_6$. However, taking extra vitamin B$_6$ can interfere with Levodopa, a medicine used to treat Parkinson's disease. See Safety Issues for more information.

Food Sources of Vitamin B$_6$

Nuts, seeds, potatoes, bananas, whole grains, and legumes are good sources of vitamin B$_6$. As we'll see, however, a typical dosage of vitamin B$_6$ supplements can be 25 or 50 times the RDA. You'd have to eat a staggering quantity of nuts and seeds to get that much vitamin B$_6$. To use vitamin B$_6$ at the higher dosages recommended for therapeutic purposes, you'd really need to take a supplement.

What Is the Scientific Evidence for Vitamin B$_6$ and Osteoporosis?

There is no direct evidence that taking high doses of B$_6$ will help prevent osteoporosis. But animal studies have found that rats deficient in vitamin B$_6$ had more fractures and slower bone-healing time.[32] In other studies, animals with B$_6$-deficient diets developed osteoporosis.[33]

Vitamin B$_6$ also promotes the breakdown of *homocysteine,* a toxic substance that is normally metabolized in the body. There is some evidence suggesting that moderate levels of homocysteine may contribute to postmenopausal bone loss.[34,35] It has been shown that supplementation with vitamin B$_6$ (especially when combined with folate) reduces high homocysteine levels in humans.[36] Given that moderate homocysteine levels may promote the development of osteoporosis, the evidence suggests that B_6 and folate may help prevent osteoporosis. However, much more research needs to be done to determine whether vitamin B_6 supplementation can really help prevent osteoporosis.

Dosage

The RDA for vitamin B_6 is 2 mg daily. We don't know what the *optimal* intake is for vitamin B_6. Much higher amounts are commonly recommended, and up to 50 mg daily appears to be safe.[37]

The basic form of vitamin B_6 is pyridoxine. In most cases, this is adequate. Vitamin B_6 must be converted to the activated form pyridoxal-5-phosphate for it to function in the body. Individuals with liver disease may not be able to make this conversion, and we recommend that anyone with liver disease speak with their primary care provider about the best way to take vitamin B_6.

Safety Issues

Vitamin B_6 is one of the few water-soluble vitamins that can be toxic to the nervous system when taken in large amounts. At higher dosages (especially above 2 g daily), the risk of nerve damage is very real. In fact, nerve-related symptoms have even been reported at doses as low as 200 mg a day.[38] Symptoms of B_6 toxicity may include tingling sensations in the feet and loss of muscle coordination.

If you are taking the tuberculosis drug isoniazid (INH) or medications for Parkinson's disease, do not take supplemental vitamin B_6 except on medical advice.

Trace Minerals

It's been known for some time that normal bone metabolism relies on several trace minerals (minerals that we need, but only in tiny amounts): manganese, boron, zinc, copper, and silicon. These trace minerals may enhance the role of calcium, and deficiencies in any of them can adversely affect bone metabolism.

One 1994 study found evidence that taking calcium plus trace mineral supplements could be more effective than calcium alone in preventing osteoporosis.[39] Fifty-nine postmenopausal women were given either (1) placebo, (2) calcium, (3) trace minerals (copper, zinc, and manganese), or (4) both calcium and trace minerals.

The group that took calcium only had no bone loss in the hip and forearm, but they did suffer spinal bone loss, although to a lesser extent than those on placebo. The women who took trace minerals alone did not experience any improvement in bone density. However, in the group of women taking calcium plus trace minerals, bone loss was stopped not only in the hip and forearm, but also in the spine. This study suggests that the combination of calcium plus trace minerals works better than calcium alone. The trace minerals alone didn't seem to help, but they seem to have made the calcium more effective.

The following sections briefly describe the relationship between these trace minerals and osteoporosis. Table 6 lists common sources of each mineral.

Manganese

Animal studies suggest that manganese is required for bone mineralization and the synthesis of connective tissue in cartilage and bone.[41]

There is also evidence that people with osteoporosis tend to be deficient in trace minerals, including manganese.[42] However, while it's clear that manganese plays a role in bone metabolism, there is no direct evidence that manganese alone is helpful in preventing osteoporosis. Good food sources include whole grains, legumes, avocados, grape juice, chocolate, seaweed, egg yolks, nuts, and

Table 6. Food Sources of Nutrients[40]

Nutrient	Common Food Sources
Magnesium	Nuts, seeds, beans, tofu, green leafy vegetables, whole grains, shrimp
Vitamin K	Green leafy vegetables, kale, parsley, spinach, broccoli, lettuce
Vitamin B_6 (Pyridoxine)	Nuts, seeds, potatoes, bananas, whole grains, legumes
Manganese	Nuts, seeds, green leafy vegetables, whole grains, dried fruit, rice bran
Boron	Kelp, sea vegetables, alfalfa, non-citrus fruits
Zinc	Shellfish, fish, red meats
Copper	Shellfish, whole grains, nuts, eggs, legumes, organ meats
Silicon	Whole grains, root vegetables

seeds. Antacids can inhibit manganese absorption, so if you take a lot of antacids, you might be low on manganese.

Safety Issues

Manganese is considered safe when taken in appropriate doses. There are reports of manganese poisoning in miners who work with this mineral in vast quantities. Early symptoms include memory loss, anxiety, mood swings, and disorientation. Neurological disorders similar to Parkinson's disease can develop. If you are taking iron, copper, zinc, magnesium, or calcium supplements, you may need extra manganese, and vice versa. In addition, if you use antacids regularly, you may also need extra manganese.

Boron

Like magnesium, boron may be essential in the conversion of vitamin D to its active form, which is needed for bone formation. Boron supplements of 3.25 mg daily have been found to increase the levels of vitamin D in the blood.[43] There is also evidence that when people whose diets are poor in boron receive boron supplements, they lose less calcium in their urine.[44] While this small study suggests that boron can help prevent osteoporosis, another more recent study failed to support these results.[45] In addition, there is some evidence that boron supplements may increase levels of estrogen in the blood,[44] so if you are receiving hormone-replacement therapy, use of boron may not be advisable.

This trace mineral is readily available through our diets and is found in many foods, including leafy vegetables, raisins, prunes, nuts, non-citrus fruits, and grains.

Safety Issues

There are no known risks from boron when taken at recommended dosages. As mentioned, it's been found to raise estrogen levels, so women already taking hormone replacement therapy (HRT) should speak with their primary care doctors before using this supplement. At extremely high doses (greater than 500 mg per day), boron can cause nausea, vomiting, and diarrhea.

Zinc

There is strong evidence that zinc plays an important role in bone metabolism, and researchers have suggested that zinc deficiency is a risk factor in the development of osteoporosis. In one small study, zinc levels were found to be low in the blood and bone of elderly patients with osteoporosis.[46] While there is no direct evidence that zinc supplementation will help prevent osteoporosis, it seems reasonable to assume that being deficient in zinc is not good for your bones.

In fact, mild zinc deficiency appears to be a common problem for many Americans.[47] Children and teenagers are especially vulnerable, since their bodies need more zinc for growth and development. Others at risk for zinc deficiency include pregnant women and the elderly, as well as those with alcoholism, sickle-cell anemia, diabetes, and kidney disease.

Oysters are a very rich source of zinc, but other food sources—seeds and nuts, peas, whole wheat, rye, and oats—are not nearly as high in zinc. There are also several forms of zinc available in supplements. Zinc picolinate, zinc citrate, and zinc acetate all seem to be efficiently absorbed. Zinc sulfate, a less expensive form, causes gastric irritation in some people.

Safety Issues

High doses of zinc (greater than 100 mg daily) taken for long periods of time can cause a number of toxic effects, including a depression of the immune system, severe copper deficiency, heart problems, and anemia.[48,49,50] If you are taking medications that reduce stomach acid such as Zantac (ranitidine) or Prilosec (omeprazole); ACE inhibitors; oral contraceptives; estrogen replacement therapy; thiazide diuretics; ethambutol; calcium; copper; or iron, you may need to take extra zinc. Use of zinc can interfere with the absorption of penicillamine and antibiotics in the tetracycline or fluoroquinolone (Cipro, Floxin) families.[51,52,53] As mentioned previously, it can also interfere with the absorption of copper, as well as magnesium and iron. Finally, the potassium-sparing diuretic amiloride was found to significantly reduce zinc excretion from the body.[54] This means that if you take zinc supplements at the same time as amiloride, zinc accumulation could occur. This could lead to toxic side effects.

Copper

Copper plays a role in the formation of connective tissue. This mineral is a cofactor in the enzyme that strengthens collagen and elastin fibers. Copper deficiency is rare, as this mineral is found in many common foods. Although some clinical and test-tube studies have suggested that copper supplements might prevent bone loss,[55,56] further research is needed before we know whether it has any real effect by itself to prevent osteoporosis. Oysters, nuts, legumes, whole grains, sweet potatoes, and dark green vegetables are good sources of copper.

Safety Issues

Copper can be toxic at high levels; copper toxicity is often due to contaminated drinking water. Symptoms include mental and physical fatigue, poor memory, depression, insomnia, nausea, vomiting, dizziness, headaches, stomach pain, and diarrhea. A characteristic metallic taste can also be noticed.

Copper is safe when taken at nutritional dosages, but these should not be exceeded. As little as 10 mg of copper daily produces nausea, and 60 mg may cause vomiting. A dose of 3.5 g or greater (over 2,000 times the recommended daily allowance) taken at one time is fatal. If you are taking zinc, iron supplements, manganese, high doses of vitamin C, ethambutol, or antacids, you may need extra copper. If you do take a copper supplement, it might be good to take it either 2 hours before or after taking these other substances.[57]

Silicon

High concentrations of silicon are found at the calcification sites of growing bone. Like copper, silicon appears to play a role in strengthening the connective tissue matrix of collagen.[58] However, like many of the minerals mentioned previously, there is no direct evidence that silicon supplements by themselves can help protect against osteoporosis. We also don't know if people can be silicon-deficient. Though there is no RDA for silicon, a daily dietary intake of 20 to 40 mg is safe and considered adequate. Unrefined grains, oatmeal, brown rice, and root vegetables are the best food sources for silicon. The herb horsetail *(Equisetum arvense)* is another rich source.

Safety Issues

A major constituent of sand, oral silicon supplements are considered nontoxic at recommended dosages.

As with any supplement, we recommend that you inform and work with your health-care provider or a nutritional expert to determine what types of supplementation will best meet your individual health needs.

Exercise, Diet, and Lifestyle: What You Can Do to Protect Your Bones

S everal natural treatments can help protect you against osteoporosis. But good health is rarely as simple as taking a vitamin or a pill. In our modern world, we are often promised quick fixes and miracle cures. But it's more realistic to see your health as the result of many different factors, including your everyday habits. Your diet, your exercise routine, your stress level, whether or not you smoke or drink heavily—these can all have a profound effect on your health. You'll get better results from any medical treatment, natural or conventional, if you also make sure your everyday habits are helping you.

This is particularly true with osteoporosis. As discussed in chapter 2, alcohol, tobacco, and possibly caffeine may increase your risk for a fracture. But one of the most important things you can do for your bones is exercise. Bones, like muscles, become stronger when you use them in vigorous exercise, and weaker when you don't use them. Bed rest can cause people to lose bone mass very rapidly—by as much as 1% per week.[1]

It's important to get enough calcium and vitamin D, as well as vitamin K and other essential nutrients. But did you know that your intake of sodium and phosphorus can also affect your bones' health? This section explains some further lifestyle changes you should make if you're concerned about osteoporosis.

Exercise

There is no better all-around support for your health than exercise. Regular, moderate exercise supports the cardiovascular system; balances your blood sugar levels; increases your strength, endurance, and lung capacity; helps you maintain a healthy weight; and boosts your emotional well-being.

Exercise also works powerfully to prevent and even reverse osteoporosis. Studies have shown that physically active people have higher bone densities than do individuals who are not active.[2] Indeed, physical inactivity is recognized as one of the factors that increases your risk for osteoporosis. The doubling rate of hip fractures in the last 30 years is thought to be partly due to our drastic decrease in physical activity.[3] Disuse, immobilization, paralysis as a result of nerve damage, or prolonged space flight (be careful before you sign up!) are all associated with marked bone loss.

There is no better all-around support for your health than exercise.

You don't have to be an athlete to benefit from regular exercise. In one recent study, 124 postmenopausal women between the ages of 50 and 70 with low bone mass performed relatively mild weight-bearing exercises (walking, stepping up and down from benches), aerobic dancing,

Gloria's Story

Gloria, a 72-year-old woman, was showering one morning when the phone rang. In her haste to answer the phone, she slipped on the wet bathroom floor and broke her hip. Gloria recovered fully from the fracture, but she was left with a psychological scar: She became terrified to walk. Having experienced one bad fall, Gloria was afraid that she might lose her balance and fall again. She began to move tentatively, touching the wall for support. Her fear kept her from regular activities.

Gloria's instincts told her to keep safe by staying still, but her inactivity was actually dangerous. Her lack of exercise, if continued, would greatly increase her risk for bone loss and more broken bones in the future. Fortunately, Gloria got help before that happened. She enrolled in a class for stretching and strengthening, and she soon regained her balance and confidence.

and flexibility exercises for 60 minutes, three times a week for a full year. At the end of the study, the women who exercised had stabilization of their spinal bone density, but the women who didn't exercise experienced a significant decrease.[4]

Several studies suggest that you can get even better results with more intense exercise. For example, one study examined the effects of intense exercises that focused on the lower forearms (near the wrists). The study participants, postmenopausal women with osteoporosis, were challenged physically in 50-minute sessions 3 times weekly over 5 months. At the end of the study period, women who exercised had an increased bone density of 3.8% while the control group continued to decline.[5]

Another study featured moderately vigorous activity (such as walking, running, playing ball games, and doing exercises on all fours) twice a week for one hour. This moderate exercise actually increased the bone mineral content of the spine in a group of healthy postmenopausal women by as much as 3 to 5% over an 8-month period. The researchers concluded that physical activity might not only stop bone loss in the lower back but also completely reverse it.[6] Remember that many of the treatments discussed here merely slow the loss of bone. The evidence that vigorous exercise can actually *reverse* bone loss is truly exciting. Exercise can also help prevent fractures indirectly, by increasing your strength and agility so that you're less likely to fall and get hurt.

What Kind of Exercise Is Best?

For preventing osteoporosis, weight-bearing exercise seems to be especially helpful. Walking, jogging, stair climbing, and other activities that place a mechanical stress on your bones (even if it's just the stress provided by your own weight) stimulate the formation of new bone.

However, other forms of exercise may be helpful as well. There is some evidence that swimming may increase bone density,[7] though we don't know for certain, because the majority of the evidence seems to come from animal studies.[8] Most studies in humans support the need for weight-bearing exercise to promote bone health.[9,10] Although swimming isn't a weight-bearing exercise, and doesn't build bone nearly as much as weight-bearing exercises do, it can be a gentle way to exercise your entire body and receive many health benefits.

In addition to the weight-bearing aerobic activities mentioned previously, resistance training (also known as weight training) ranks high in importance for helping to prevent osteoporosis.[11] Dr. Tim Lohman, Professor of

Physiology at the University of Arizona's College of Medicine, is the principal researcher conducting a 4-year study on resistance training (i.e., weight lifting or using an exercise machine) and postmenopausal bone loss. Dr. Lohman recommends a regimen of vigorous resistance training that involves six to eight repetitions in each major muscle group, especially those that affect the hip and back. The repetitions, Dr. Lohman says, must be difficult enough to leave your muscles fatigued at the end of the set.

Don't plunge into an intense new exercise program; it's much better (and safer) to gradually increase your activity.

In choosing a type of exercise for yourself, you might want to consult with your doctor or other health care provider. Don't plunge into an intense new exercise program; it's much better (and safer) to gradually increase your activity. And try to choose a form of exercise that you enjoy, because to get its benefits, you'll need to keep doing it, week after week.

How Much Should You Exercise?

In the studies discussed previously, bone loss was stopped or reversed by an exercise regimen of 1 hour 2 to 3 times a week. For optimal effects on your bones, we recommend that you exercise four or five times per week for at least 30 minutes of weight-bearing exercise, plus at least 2 times per week of weight resistance exercise. If you can exercise daily, that's even better.

However, we understand that this can be a rather aggressive schedule. Again, a minimum of 2 days of exercise seems necessary to protect bone health, but any exercise regimen is better than none—for a whole host of health reasons! A qualified health-care practitioner can determine what will work best for you after analyzing your age, past exercise level, and current health status.

Regular exercise keeps you in shape so that you're less likely to hurt yourself, the way you might if you only occasionally attempt an intense workout. You're more likely to injure yourself if you plunge into an intensive exercise program before you're in shape for it. Injury can also be the result of beginning vigorous exercise before your muscles have warmed up, so be sure to begin each session with at least 5–10 minutes of light walking or jogging to get your muscles ready.

For optimal effects on your bones, we recommend that you exercise four or five times per week for at least 30 minutes of weight-bearing exercise, plus at least 2 times per week of weight resistance exercise.

The intensity of exercise you choose should fit your general health level. If you have cardiovascular disease or other health conditions that might affect your ability to exercise safely, you should consult your doctor before you begin a new exercise program or change your exercise habits.

Premenopausal women have an additional risk in over-exercising. As you may remember from chapters 2 and 3, some women exercise (and diet) so intensely that their bodies can no longer produce enough estrogen and progesterone, and they stop menstruating. When this happens, the consequences can be severe: infertility and rapid loss of bone. Premenopausal women who have stopped menstruating because of intense exercise and dieting need to cut back on the intensity of training and improve their diet to raise their body fat to a healthier level.

Salt: Sodium and Calcium Don't Mix

Although the body requires only about 500 mg (about ¼ teaspoon) of sodium per day to function properly, one review reported that the majority of people living in developed countries ate anywhere from 10 to 35 times that amount.[12] More recently, the American Dietetic Association estimated that adults in the U.S. consume around 4,000 to 6,000 mg of salt per day, 2 to 3 teaspoons' worth![13] Table salt and processed foods are our main sources of sodium, an important nutrient that most of us consume excessively.

Table salt and processed foods are our main sources of sodium, an important nutrient that most of us consume excessively.

Why the focus on salt? Well, you probably know that too much sodium can raise blood pressure for some people, but do you know that it can also cause your body to lose calcium? When you eat more sodium than your body needs, you eliminate the extra sodium through your kidneys. This extra sodium prevents your kidneys from hanging onto the calcium in your blood, and so calcium gets swept out with the sodium. In addition to the calcium that's lost in the urine when salt is excreted from the body, researchers have also noted compounds related to bone resorption. This was observed in one small study, which showed that young women who increased their dietary intake of salt had increased levels of calcium and another compound related to bone breakdown in their urine.[14] In another study,

How to Cut Your Salt Intake in Half

If you are like most Americans, you may be eating a lot of canned and frozen food, and you go to restaurants fairly often. You love spicy foods like salsa and pizza, and you also enjoy the occasional snack of chips, olives, or pickles. Your sodium intake may be as high as 3,000 to 4,000 mg a day.

You can easily cut your salt intake in half by following these simple guidelines:

- When buying pre-prepared food, look at the sodium content listed on the label. Choose products with less than 300 mg per serving.
- When eating out, try to avoid casseroles, soups, creamed dishes, and sauces. Very often these can add up to 3,000 mg of sodium in a single meal.
- Whenever possible, use fresh foods instead of processed ones. This is the best way to control how much salt goes into your food. And fresh fruits and vegetables are healthier for you in other ways as well.
- Finally, go easy on the salt shaker. Try low-sodium seasonings instead.

researchers looked at how salt in the diet affected bone density in 124 postmenopausal women receiving either calcium supplementation or placebo. Interestingly, researchers did not alter the women's salt intake in any way; that is, women ate as much salt as they might normally eat in their diets. Because of the challenge of measuring how much salt each woman was eating (from a diet diary), salt intake was estimated by how much salt was eliminated in the urine. The study showed two things: (1) High salt intake in the diet (as estimated by salt in the urine) was associated with an increase in bone loss in the hip, and (2) increasing calcium in the diet protected against bone loss in the hip.

In addition, the researchers noted that salt had an important effect on calcium in the diet and on bone density in these women. When the amount of salt eliminated in the urine (the measure of how much salt the women were eating) was cut in half (reduced from nearly 3,500 mg to 1,700 mg), the result was a beneficial effect on bone density, as if the women had increased their daily intake of calcium by 900 mg.[15] *The bottom line:* Ease up on the shaker and watch the salt content of your foods. Although it may be a little jarring to your taste buds initially, given the multitude of health benefits you can get from cutting down on sodium, it's a good thing to do.

Phosphorus and Calcium: A Question of Balance

Phosphorus, like calcium, is an important mineral in bone. Bone crystals contain both phosphorus and calcium. But while most of us get too little calcium, the opposite is true for phosphorus: The American diet often provides too much.

When you get much more phosphorus than calcium, it can cause elevations of PTH (parathyroid hormone), a hormone that can cause calcium to be removed from bone. Parathyroid hormone is essential for maintaining the proper level of vitamin D in the body, which you may remember is calcium's partner in assuring bone health.

Processed foods and soft drinks are a major source of phosphorus in our diets. Soft drinks alone account for about 25% of the phosphorus in the typical American diet. Cola drinks contain up to 500 mg per 12-ounce can! The impact of our diets on our bones' health cannot be emphasized too strongly. Research in children and adolescents suggests that an imbalance of phosphorus and calcium may be associated with an increase in the risk of fractures. A study of 127 younger boys and girls (ages 8 to 16) found that girls with low ratios of dietary calcium to phosphorus had more bone fractures.[16] And girls who drank cola beverages (more than one per day) were more than three times as likely to break a bone. The boys who drank a lot of cola did not show the same increase in fractures, but their calcium intake was significantly higher than the girls'.

Research in young adults has also raised concern about the impact of an imbalance between calcium and phosphorous in the diet. For example, a study of college-age men showed how closely related the levels of phosphorous and levels of vitamin D are in the body.[17] High-phosphorus diets have been linked to lower bone density in the wrist in women aged 24 to 28.[18]

In addition, studies have found high PTH levels in young women (aged 18 to 25) whose diets supplied a low ratio of calcium to phosphorus.[19,20] The researchers voiced concern that the typical diet of young women might negatively affect the balance between bone building and bone breakdown at a critical period of their bone growth. (You may remember that our peak bone mass is reached sometime between 20 and 30 years of age, making our late teens to early 20s a critical period of bone growth.) Because women aged 16 to 25 years and older have the greatest calcium-phosphorus imbalances, and because optimal dietary intake of bone-building nutrients early in life may be the best way to prevent or delay osteoporosis, this is an issue that deserves some real attention.[21]

So, what about the effects of phosphorous in the diet on osteoporosis? The issue is not as clear-cut as one might

Table 7. Phosphorus and Sodium Content of Typical Foods[23]

Food	Calcium (mg)/ Phosphorus (mg)	Sodium (mg)
Large cheeseburger	273/411	1,666
Large cheese dog	297/312	1,986
Pizza, ½ of 12-inch round	518/529	1,347
Mexican style frozen dinner	154/386	1,793
Chicken, 3½ oz, roasted	15/216	77
Picante sauce, 6 tablespoons	18/60	480
Hamburger, lean	14/233	41
Large pickle, sour	21/26	1,428
Olives, Greek (3 of medium size)	0/6	658

expect. In older women who have osteoporosis, researchers have been trying to understand the complex balance between parathyroid hormone (PTH), vitamin D levels in the body, and the effect of phosphorous. Some research that evaluated the effects of a large dose of phosphate on women with osteoporosis showed that they were not able to make as much PTH as needed to maintain vitamin D levels in their blood.[22] However, whether the same response would occur if women ingested a normal amount of phosphorous in their diet is unclear. As you might expect, this abnormal response (lower PTH production and inability to maintain adequate vitamin D levels) to a high dose of phosphate in women with osteoporosis is of concern, since vitamin D is needed for bone formation and many elderly women (and men) are already deficient in vitamin D. Despite these findings, we are not completely certain how normal dietary phosphorus intake affects osteoporosis. From the evidence we have today, it makes sense to try to keep your intake of calcium and phosphorus in balance. For most of us, this means getting more calcium and less phosphorus (see table 7). Cutting back on soda (especially cola) and fast food will cut your intake of phosphorus.

Progesterone: An Option for Osteoporosis?

P rogesterone is a key hormone of a woman's reproductive health. In the first half of a woman's menstrual cycle, the ovaries produce progesterone,
which causes the uterus to get ready to receive and nourish a fertilized egg. If none appears, the progesterone
level falls and menstruation begins. Progesterone also
plays important roles throughout pregnancy: Without
enough of this hormone, a woman would not be able to
carry a child to birth.

As with estrogen, menopause leads to a dramatic drop
in the body's level of progesterone. But while we have at
least some understanding of the effects of estrogen loss,
less is known about progesterone. Today, progesterone (or
a chemical equivalent of it) is used routinely to reduce
certain health risks involved in taking estrogen after
menopause. However, it has not been fully established
whether or not progesterone may play a more direct role
in protecting against osteoporosis.

Progesterone and Menopause

In the mid 1970s, the *New England Journal of Medicine* published three disturbing reports regarding estrogen replacement therapy, which had become popular in the late 1960s. These reports found a four- to five-fold increase in the risk of uterine cancer among women who had taken estrogen.[1,2]

During a woman's menstrual cycle, estrogen and progesterone orchestrate the buildup and shedding of the uterine lining, which prepares itself each month to nourish a fertilized egg. After menopause, this cycle stops. But if a woman takes supplemental estrogen after menopause, her uterine lining may build up as before, without shedding. This tissue buildup contributes to a higher risk for uterine cancer.

Because of this risk, the recommended approach is to give HRT (estrogen with progesterone or a chemical with a very similar effect to progesterone) rather than just ERT (estrogen alone) to women who have an intact uterus and could therefore get uterine cancer. The added progesterone ensures that the uterine lining sheds, thereby effectively preventing the buildup of the uterine lining. (This means, by the way, that a postmenopausal woman taking these hormones may continue to have monthly "periods.") In fact, one scientific review stated that when given for 10 days each month, progestins (chemicals similar to progesterone) are 98% effective in reversing the overgrowth of the lining of the uterus.[3] Numerous other studies support the role that progestins play in reversing endometrial overgrowth as well.[4]

Studies have confirmed that taking progesterone with estrogen all but eliminates the health risk for endometrial cancer. That is, a woman who takes HRT instead of just ERT has about the same risk for cancer of the uterus as a woman who takes no hormones.

Much of the "progesterone" used in conventional hormone replacement therapy is actually progestins, laboratory-synthesized "chemical cousins" of progesterone. In addition to protecting women on estrogen therapy against uterine cancer, there is growing evidence that progesterone or progestins offer other benefits during menopause. Progesterone appears to reduce hot flashes and improve blood lipid profiles (both HDL ["good"] and LDL ["bad"] cholesterol), although the evidence for these effects is less well established than for estrogen. However, some progestins, such as norethindrone, *decrease* estrogen's effectiveness at improving blood lipid profiles.[5] Although there has been some preliminary research suggesting that progestational agents may decrease the risk of breast cancer, the evidence is mixed.[6] In fact, two recent studies give reasonably strong evidence that the use of estrogen and progestins together (HRT) puts women at a substantially higher risk for breast cancer than the use of estrogen (ERT) alone.[7,8]

Studies have confirmed that taking progesterone with estrogen all but eliminates the health risk for endometrial cancer.

These findings have important ramifications regarding the use of hormone therapy. A word of caution: If you are currently taking HRT, do not abruptly stop taking your current therapy. It is critical that you speak with your health-care provider about determining which regimen will be the healthiest and safest one for you.

Progesterone vs. Progestins

Until fairly recently, there was a problem with taking progesterone: It couldn't be taken orally, because the process of digestion destroyed it. Women could take prog-esterone in the form of a skin cream or suppository, but many women wanted a less messy, more convenient form. For this reason, pharmaceutical companies developed the

progestins, synthetic chemicals that were very similar to proges-terone, but could be taken in a pill (see table 8).

If you are currently taking HRT, do not abruptly stop taking your current therapy.

Though the progestins' chem-ical structures are similar to prog-esterone's (see figure 8), there seem to be significantly different effects in the body.[9] Many women experience uncomfort-able side effects with progestins. The differences in the chemical

structures of progesterone and synthetic progestins are slight, but the effect in the body is significant. The prog-estins, especially one called norethindrone, cause women to retain more sodium and water in their bodies, leading to bloating. Many women have other side effects when taking progestins, including breast tenderness, weight gain, men-tal depression, nausea, insomnia, headaches, acne, and skin rash. These side effects can be enough to discourage a woman from taking hormone replacement therapy.

Today, another choice is available. *Micronized prog-esterone* is a form of progesterone that can be taken orally. Unlike the progestins, micronized progesterone is chemically identical to the natural progesterone your body produces. It is "true" progesterone, not just a chemical with a similar effect. This true progesterone may be a better alternative for women who experience side effects from progestins. Micronized progesterone has been shown to be effective for postmenopausal hor-mone replacement therapy (HRT), as well as for other

Table 8. Oral Progestins Currently Available

Generic Name	Trade Name	Dosage (mg)	Manu- facturer
Medroxy- progesterone acetate	Provera	2.5–10	Upjohn
Medroxy- progesterone acetate	Curretab	10	Reid- Provident
Medroxy- progesterone acetate	Amen	10	Carnrick
Norethindrone	Norlutin	5	Parke-Davis
Norethindrone	Micronor	0.35	Ortho
Norethindrone	Nor-Q-D	0.35	Syntex
Norethindrone acetate	Norlutate	5	Parke-Davis
Norgestrel	Ovrette	0.075	Wyeth

conditions such as premenstrual syndrome, premature labor, and to replace the progesterone production of absent ovaries.[10–14]

However, the evidence has not been uniformly positive. One double-blind placebo-controlled study of 185 women with PMS found that oral micronized progesterone was no better than placebo for the treatment of severe symptoms.[15]

So what's the bottom line here? While some evidence suggests that true progesterone may be a reasonable alternative to progestin for a variety of uses, more research needs to be done, especially regarding its effects on bone.

Progestins, Natural Progesterone, and Bone

As we've mentioned, estrogen protects bone by blocking the breakdown of bone tissue by cells called osteoclasts.

> While some evidence suggests that true progesterone may be a reasonable alternative to progestin for a variety of uses, more research needs to be done, especially regarding its effects on bone.

However, some researchers have suggested that the progestins may do something different to help bone: They may increase bone formation.[16,17] Though it's not clear exactly how they work, some evidence suggests that progestins may be effective by themselves in preventing the postmenopausal bone loss that leads to osteoporosis.

For example, in one small study, 36 postmenopausal women were divided into three groups. They were given Provera (a progestin), estrogen alone, or a combination of both for 18 months. No significant differences in bone mass were detected in the three treatment groups. (A slight increase, too small to be statistically significant, was noted in women taking the combined therapy.) The results of this study would seem to indicate that progestins may work as well as estrogen at slowing bone loss, although larger studies are needed to confirm whether progestins by themselves have any positive effect on bone.[18]

And what about natural progesterone's effects on bone? Unfortunately, not much research has been completed in this area. However, one recent study looked at

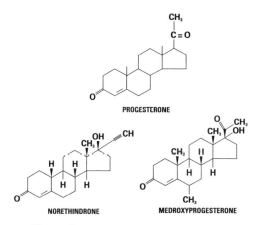

Figure 8. *Progesterone vs. progestins*

the effectiveness of natural progesterone cream on bone loss, as well as hot flashes, in 102 healthy women in their early postmenopausal years. The women applied either the cream or placebo to their skin daily and were evaluated after one year. Although they showed definite improvement in hot flashes, no protective effect on bone was noted.[19]

While the preliminary evidence that progestins may help against bone loss may appear to be good news for breast cancer survivors and other women who can't take estrogen, the issue is far from settled. At least one large observational study found that progestins alone may raise the risk for breast cancer.[20]

Again, until more definitive evidence is available to tell us about the positive or negative effects of progesterone and progestins taken by themselves, we highly encourage you to speak with your health care provider to determine which therapies are best for you.

Progesterone: Better Than Estrogen?

If you've read books or articles about natural treatments for osteoporosis, you may have heard the theory that progesterone fights osteoporosis. According to this theory, progesterone is as crucial for protecting postmenopausal women's bone mass as estrogen—or even more so.

Much more research needs to be done on this question.

Progesterone Taken Alone

Many women cannot take estrogen therapy because their medical history makes estrogen too risky. Women who have, or have had, cancer of the uterus or breast, hypertension, diabetes, liver disease, or thrombophlebitis (inflammation of a vein associated with a blood clot) are advised not to take estrogen. (See chapter 9 for further information about estrogen replacement therapy.)

There are also some women who react strongly to even small dosages of estrogen. Undesirable symptoms such as breast tenderness, worsening of fibrocystic disease, breakthrough bleeding, and growth of uterine fibroid tumors have been reported by women on estrogen therapy.

Women who can't take estrogen may benefit by using progesterone alone. There is some evidence that progesterone, taken alone, can reduce hot flashes. It also seems to improve blood lipid profiles (that is, the ratio of "good" to "bad" cholesterol in the blood), though further research needs to done on progesterone's ability to protect against cardiovascular disease. Based on his own research, Dr. John Lee, an obstetrician/gynecologist, has suggested a therapy of progesterone taken alone to treat the symptoms of menopause and reverse bone loss. He recom-

Lori's Story

Lori, a 39-year-old mother of three, had just given birth to twins when she began having hot flashes, night sweats, and other menopausal symptoms. At first it was difficult for her to tell whether her symptoms were related to recently giving birth, the demands of caring for the children, or the significant decline of her hormones. Lori was told she was too young to be entering menopause, but after several months and a lot of reading, she asked to have a blood test (FSH and LH) done (this test can determine whether a woman has entered menopause).

Lori's test results confirmed that she was indeed menopausal. She was advised to take HRT in the form of Premarin and Provera, which she began with the hope that her symptoms would be alleviated. But the side effects of the progestin (Provera) left her wondering whether she was any better off (she was experiencing severe headaches, weight gain, and depression). Luckily, she was able to switch to a micronized progesterone, which allowed her to keep the benefits of hormone replacement therapy without the side effects of the progestin.

mends applying progesterone to the skin in the form of a cream. However, his research has been sharply criticized for being too scanty and poorly designed to provide meaningful results.[21] As mentioned previously, one recent study that looked at the effects of progesterone skin cream on bone showed no protective benefit.[19]

Clearly, much more research is needed to determine whether it is really better to use progesterone alone instead of in combination with estrogen. At the present time, estrogen's benefits and risks are much more

"Natural" Progesterone vs. Progestins

If you read books or magazines about natural medicine, you may have heard that "natural" progesterone is better than the "synthetic" variety. What do these terms mean?

Actually, the difference is a bit confusing. Often, when a substance is called "natural," it means that it has been extracted, with minimal processing, from a natural source such as a plant. But so-called "natural" progesterone is made in a laboratory. The reason it's called "natural" is that it's chemically identical to the biological hormone made in the body. "Natural" isn't really the right word for it, though. We'll call this form "true" progesterone, because it is exactly the same as your body's own progesterone.

True progesterone's chemical cousins, the progestins, are made in a laboratory, and thus are a bit different from the natural hormone your body produces.

solidly established. Check with your physician for the latest information.

Dosage

Progestins are available only by prescription. Typically, a progestin such as Provera (in a dosage ranging from 2.5 to 10 mg daily) is given for 7 to 14 days each month. Consult your physician for dosage information (see table 9).

Micronized progesterone is available without a prescription. However, we strongly recommend medical supervision. It can be taken in many ways:

The marketing of a variety of "natural" progesterone products, however, has made things a bit more complicated. There have been claims that the wild yam plant contains natural progesterone. In fact, there is no progesterone in the wild yam. This plant contains a chemical called *diosgenin,* which is a chemical precursor of progesterone; our bodies cannot convert diosgenin from wild yams into progesterone, so taking wild yam won't raise your progesterone levels. Because of this, some manufacturers add small amounts of true progesterone to wild yam creams. Check the label, or consult a nutritionally oriented health-care provider for guidance on wild yam products.

- *Capsules* of oral progesterone are typically taken in dosages of 100 to 200 mg daily. There is no specific evidence as to the best dosage. You and your health-care provider can monitor the effects of various dosages, using blood tests when appropriate.
- *Sublingual* drops are placed under the tongue and held there for a few minutes. The drops are absorbed rapidly through the mucus membranes in the mouth; however, the levels of progesterone fall in 3 to 4 hours as the drops are rapidly metabolized. The dosage (number of drops) varies with the product, so you'll need to follow the directions on the label.

Table 9. Equivalent Dosages: Provera and Progesterone

Provera	Micronized Progesterone (Oral)
10 mg per day	100 mg 2 times per day
5 mg per day	50 mg 2 times per day
2.5 mg per day	25 mg 2 times per day

- **Transdermal** means "through the skin." Transdermal progesterone comes in skin creams and oils. **Note:** Creams that contain progesterone will not be as effective if the product is suspended in mineral oil. Other products, depending on the shelf life, may deteriorate over time with oxygen exposure. It may be better to buy a progesterone cream that comes in a tube rather than a jar, because of the reduced exposure to oxygen. Also, the cream or oil needs to be potent enough to have an effect. Amounts below 800 mg per 2-ounce jar will not supply enough progesterone if you do not produce enough progesterone. If you use one of these products, you should consider consulting your health-care provider, who can order the proper blood tests to confirm appropriate treatment levels.

Safety Issues

The progestins are associated with several uncomfortable side effects, including water retention, breast tenderness, weight gain, depression, nausea, insomnia, headaches, acne, and skin rash. Also, taking progestins can lower your body's production of its own progesterone.[22]

Micronized progesterone is thought to produce fewer side effects, though it has been slightly associated with an

Esther's and Kathy's Stories

Esther, a 62-year-old woman who had entered menopause 15 years prior, was still having monthly bleeding. Her concern about heart disease and osteoporosis led her to choose hormone replacement therapy (HRT); however, the progestin she took caused her to continue having monthly "periods." She wasn't happy with this situation, but she preferred to put up with the inconvenience rather than discontinue the HRT.

Kathy felt differently. She decided to remove herself from HRT after being on it for 2 years. She said that the side effects were intolerable, especially the continued monthly bleeding. This sentiment is shared by many women.

increased incidence of blood clots, and at doses of 400 mg or greater is reportedly associated with drowsiness. Micronized progesterone's safety has not yet been studied thoroughly enough to establish conclusively that it's safer than progestins. Consult your health-care provider for the latest information on progestins (especially regarding their use in HRT and breast cancer) and micronized progesterone. An unpopular feature of both progestins and true progesterone is that most women who take either one continue to have monthly periods. In fact, the majority of postmenopausal women who take estrogen plus a progestin continue to have some type of cyclical uterine bleeding well into old age.

Many women dislike the continued monthly bleeding cycle after they've gone through menopause. Monthly periods may not be necessary, however, with daily doses of micronized progesterone and estradiol. Dr. Joel Hargrove, a researcher at Harvard University, has conducted trials with daily oral micronized estrogen and progesterone. In one study, postmenopausal women who received micronized progesterone (200–300 mg) along with 0.5 mg of estradiol on a continuous daily basis did not menstruate. Significantly, this lack of bleeding was not associated with any buildup of the uterine lining.[23] Other research using micronized progesterone has shown similar findings.[24]

Conventional Treatments for Osteoporosis

T here are several effective conventional medications for osteoporosis. These can be used alone or combined with natural approaches such as exercise, nutritional supplements, natural hormone therapy, and diet. You and your health care provider can consider all the options and then decide which approach fits you best (see table 10).

For years, hormone replacement therapy (HRT) has been the leading medical approach to preventing postmenopausal osteoporosis. This section discusses estrogen replacement therapy (ERT) and hormone replacement therapy. (Remember, HRT is simply ERT plus an equivalent of progesterone.) We'll look at these therapies' advantages and risks to help you and your doctor decide whether hormone therapy is right for you. We'll also look at the other most important osteoporosis medications available today, including alendronate (Fosamax), calcitonin, and raloxifene (Evista).

Table 10. Conventional Treatments for Osteoporosis

Medication	Indications	Effective Dosage	Risk Factors	Side Effects
Estrogen	Prevention and treatment	0.625 mg daily (Premarin and Ogen) 1 mg daily (Estradiol) 0.05 mg transdermal patch (Estraderm)	Breast cancer Uterine cancer Gallbladder disease Abnormal blood clots	Breast tenderness Fluid retention Mood disturbances Weight gain Headaches Acne
Progesterone (used with estrogen)	Prevention and treatment	2.5–10 mg daily (Provera) 100 mg daily of natural progesterone	Possible increase in breast cancer risk	Irregular menstrual bleeding Fluid retention Mood disturbances Weight gain
Alendronate (Fosamax)	Prevention and treatment	10 mg daily	Esophageal ulcers	Heartburn Constipation Diarrhea Bloating, gas

Table 10. Conventional Treatments for Osteoporosis (continued)

Medication	Indications	Effective Dosage	Risk Factors	Side Effects
Raloxifene (Evista)	Prevention	60 mg daily	Deep vein thrombosis	Hot flashes Leg cramps
Calcitonin	Treatment	200 IU daily	Secondary hyperparathyroidism Anti-CT antibody production	Injectable: nausea, vomiting, vertigo Intranasal: rhinitis, nasal irritation
Tamoxifen	Prevention	20 mg daily	Uterine and liver cancer	Menstrual irregularities Visual impairment
Sodium fluoride	Prevention	40–80 mg daily	Weakening of bones GI bleeding	Anemia Nausea Inflamed joints

Estrogen Replacement Therapy

By now, you're most likely quite aware that there's an important link between menopause and osteoporosis. After menopause, a woman may begin to lose bone mass rapidly for 3 to 6 years, leaving her much more vulnerable to osteoporosis.

As discussed in chapter 3, the main reason for this bone loss is thought to be the sudden drop in the body's estrogen levels. Some experts consider that a certain amount of a woman's bone mass is "estrogen-dependent," meaning that she gains it after puberty and loses it when her estrogen levels fall in menopause. Estrogen protects women's bones by inhibiting the activity of *osteoclasts*, the cells that break down and resorb bone. See chapter 3 for more information about the relationship between estrogen, menopause, and osteoporosis.

Estrogen replacement therapy (ERT) and hormone replacement therapy (HRT) have been the cornerstone of medical treatments to prevent osteoporosis, and their effectiveness has been proven in numerous clinical studies. The evidence from prospective as well as retrospective studies shows that estrogen, when taken in adequate dosages and within 5 years of menopause, can prevent and perhaps partially reverse bone loss and reduce fractures of the hip, wrist, and spine. In general, long-term estrogen use appears to reduce the risk of fracture by about 50%.[1]

Estrogen's effect on bone varies in different parts of the skeleton. For example, within 2 years of starting estrogen, there is a small but significant increase in bone mineral density in the lumbar (lower) spine. It seems to take even longer—at least 5 years—for significant results to appear in the hip.

Several studies have concluded that estrogen replacement therapy provides significant protection of bone only when it's taken for the long term.[2] If a woman stops taking

Forms of Estrogen

The most common form of estrogen given to postmenopausal women is called "conjugated equine estrogen," or Premarin. This form of estrogen is taken from the urine of pregnant horses. Although it is a natural source, there are many who find the harvesting of pregnant horses' urine for human usage definitely unnatural. (Horse estrogens don't precisely match human estrogen.)

There are different forms in which estrogen can be taken: orally as a pill, or through the skin by means of a patch. A purely synthetic form of estrogen is also available.

estrogen after only 5 or 10 years, there is a risk that she may begin to lose bone rapidly. It appears that in order to keep the bone-protecting benefits of postmenopausal estrogen, a woman must keep taking it.[2]

Advantages of Estrogen Replacement Therapy

There is no question that taking estrogen significantly protects against bone loss. It is also thought to have other health benefits for postmenopausal women. Most immediately, it relieves hot flashes, vaginal dryness, and other uncomfortable symptoms of menopause.

It has been observed that taking estrogen often has a positive effect on mood and behavior. The precise mode of action is not known, but it is believed that estrogen may modify the metabolism of the neurotransmitters in the brain. It has been suggested that estrogen may help prevent or delay Alzheimer's disease, but the studies on which this idea is based are highly preliminary.

Estrogen is frequently said to offer considerable protection against cardiovascular disease, the leading cause of death for women over age 50 in the United States. However, the scientific research on this subject is actually much less convincing than is often reported. Most of the evidence comes from observational studies, a type of study that can be quite misleading, since it cannot prove cause-and-effect relationships. The only double-blind study reported thus far on the subject was controversial: Although it found a beneficial heart effect in women who had been taking HRT for several years, it found no overall heart benefit for women during the early years of taking HRT.[3] In fact, the women who took HRT had significantly more cases of gallbladder disease and thromboembolism (blood clots) than did the placebo group.

Safety Issues

Although estrogen replacement therapy has been widely used for decades, there are still many things we don't know about its safety. The Women's Health Initiative, the largest study on this subject to date, is looking at the effects of HRT, diet, and lifestyle modifications on cardiovascular disease, cancer risk, and osteoporosis. This major study, conducted by the National Institutes of Health, should answer many of our questions. Very preliminary data from this trial indicate that women may have more cardiovascular problems during their first two years of using estrogen. However, researchers have cautioned that this early information is not significant enough to alter current medical practices. Unfortunately, a definitive answer is not expected to be available until 2005. In the meantime, we can only present what we know today about the risks and side effects of estrogen.

Breast Cancer

Approximately 10% of all women in the United States will develop breast cancer in their lifetime. Although the evidence isn't consistent, two major studies have found that estrogen replacement therapy increased certain groups' risk for breast cancer by 50% or more.[4] Specifically, the risk was most pronounced in women who were older than 55 and who had been using a hormone therapy (estrogen alone or estrogen plus a progestin) for more than 5 years. More recently, a third major study has found evidence that estrogen primarily increases the risk of relatively uncommon types of breast cancer that usually respond well to treatment.[5] Even so, any increase in a woman's risk for breast cancer is worrisome.

The question of estrogen and breast cancer remains controversial.

The question of estrogen and breast cancer remains controversial. While major studies have found evidence of some kind of link, other studies have failed to find any relationship. Given the concerns of women and health practitioners alike, more research is clearly needed and is underway. It's possible that low-dose and/or short-term (less than 5 years) use of ERT/HRT does not substantially increase the risk of breast cancer.[6] However, women usually need to take estrogen for much longer than 5 years—probably indefinitely—in order to get substantial, lasting protection against osteoporosis.[7]

Some medical authorities hold that, while estrogen may increase the risk of breast cancer, its benefits for cardiovascular disease more than outweigh this risk. However, as mentioned previously, we don't yet know for sure that estrogen prevents cardiovascular disease.[8]

In any case, if you have breast cancer, or have had it in the past, you should definitely avoid estrogen. Many types of breast cancer are accelerated by estrogen therapy, and there is good reason to believe that ERT/HRT may increase the overall rate of recurrence among women who have already had breast cancer.[9]

Cancer of the Uterus (Endometrial Cancer)

Cancer of the uterine lining (endometrium) is the fourth most common cancer among women in the United States.[9] Since 1975, nearly two dozen reports have confirmed that ERT significantly increases a woman's risk for endometrial cancer. Recent studies have shown that the increased risk remains for up to 15 years after discontinuing estrogen.[9] This risk can be significantly reduced or eliminated by adding progesterone or a progestin for 7 or more days per month. For this reason, the recommended approach is to give HRT rather than just ERT to women who have an intact uterus and could therefore get uterine cancer.

Women who already have a uterine fibroid tumor are usually not given ERT, because it can increase the tumor's size.

Gallbladder Disease

Women who use ERT or HRT are twice as likely to develop gallbladder disease needing surgery than women who do not take estrogen.[10]

Abnormal Blood Clots

You may already know that oral contraceptives can increase a woman's risk for thromboembolism (the blockage of a blood vessel by a blood clot). Taking estrogen may also increase this risk, although probably to a lesser extent.

Side Effects of Estrogen (ERT) and HRT

In addition to the serious health risks we've just looked at, women also report a number of annoying side effects when they take estrogen, including breast tenderness, weight gain, headache, bloating, and fluid retention. Some of these side effects may be related to too high a dosage of estrogen and might be relieved by reducing the dosage. Varying the progesterone dosage might help as well.

When Not to Take Estrogen

Estrogen is generally not recommended for women with certain medical conditions, including:

- Pregnancy (known or suspected)
- Breast cancer (previously diagnosed or suspected estrogen-dependent breast cancer, certain types of breast cancer known to be affected by estrogen)
- Cancer of the uterus or endometrium (uterine lining)
- Unexplained abnormal uterine bleeding
- Uterine fibroid tumors
- History of blood clot formation (thrombosis)
- Active liver disease

Raloxifene (Evista)

Raloxifene (trade name Evista) is a drug that was recently approved for the prevention of osteoporosis. It is one of a new class of drugs called Selective Estrogen Receptor Modulators (SERMs). As the search for improved estrogen-like medications continues, the SERMs will undoubtedly take the spotlight.

The SERMs are designed to behave like estrogen in some parts of the body but not others. In particular, they do not appear to affect the breast and uterus, and therefore should not increase the risk of cancer in these areas. One particular SERM, raloxifene, seems to help prevent certain types of breast cancer.[11]

However, the SERMs' full range of risks and side effects may not be known for several years. Ongoing research and long-term clinical studies must continue. For the present, raloxifene may be considered for women who cannot or should not take estrogen, yet are at high risk for osteoporosis.

Benefits of Raloxifene

Raloxifene is designed to prevent bone loss and has been found to build bone density. It has also been found to reduce the risk of spinal fracture in postmenopausal women with osteoporosis.[12] In addition, it may reduce blood levels of harmful forms of cholesterol. And it seems to do all this without increasing the risk of cancer in the breast or uterus.

However, raloxifene seems to be not quite as helpful as estrogen in certain respects. For example, it doesn't relieve menopausal symptoms such as hot flashes or vaginal dryness. Also, while estrogen is thought to improve levels of HDL ("good") cholesterol, raloxifene seems to have no such effect. On the other hand, raloxifene doesn't cause the side effects associated with estrogen and HRT, such as breast tenderness or menstrual bleeding.

Safety Issues

Like estrogen, a clear health risk associated with raloxifene thus far is deep venous thrombosis, a condition in which blood clots form in the blood vessels. The most common minor side effect of raloxifene appears to be leg cramps, experienced by 6% of women who use it. And if you transition from estrogen to raloxifene, you may develop menopausal symptoms such as hot flashes.

The biggest concern with raloxifene is the possibility that it might increase the rate of certain forms of cancer. Large-scale studies of raloxifene are presently underway and should help clearly define its risks and benefits.

Bisphosphonates

Bisphosphonates are a group of compounds that, somewhat like estrogen, prevent bone loss by interfering with the action of the *osteoclasts* (the cells that break down, or *resorb*, bone). Bisphosphonates bind to osteoclasts and reduce their rate of activity. Unlike estrogen, these drugs also work on calcium phosphate crystals in bone directly, preventing them from dissolving.

The U.S. Food and Drug Administration recently approved alendronate (Fosamax), a bisphosphonate, for the prevention and treatment of osteoporosis.

Benefits of Alendronate (Fosamax)

Alendronate has been marketed as an alternative to estrogen in the fight against osteoporosis. It effectively decreases or even reverses bone loss in postmenopausal women, without the side effects and risks associated with ERT. Studies have shown that, taken over a 3-year period, alendronate decreases spinal fractures by 48% and increases bone density by about 5 to 10%.[13]

Safety Issues

The worst side effect of alendronate involves stomach problems. Unless it's taken in a very specific way, it can cause severe ulcers in the esophagus. Alendronate must be taken on an empty stomach with 8 ounces of water immediately after waking in the morning, at least one-half hour before any food, drink, or other medications. In one study, participants were instructed to stay in an upright position for at least 60 minutes after taking alendronate so that the pill could be fully absorbed.[14] Many users find a regimen like this annoying and complex, and it is one of the more common reasons given for discontinuing the medication.

Alendronate can also cause other gastrointestinal side effects, including abdominal pain, nausea, heartburn, difficulty swallowing, bloating, gas, constipation, and diarrhea.

Calcitonin

Calcitonin is a hormone produced by the thyroid gland that occurs naturally in the body. As a powerful inhibitor of *osteoclasts* (the cells that resorb bone), calcitonin slows the rate of bone breakdown, much as ERT and alendronate do. Calcitonin has been approved for treating osteoporosis since late 1984.

Benefits of Calcitonin

Calcitonin slows bone loss and increases bone density in the spine and the rest of the body. Some patients report that it also relieves the pain associated with bone fractures. Studies suggest a possible explanation for this: calcitonin triggers the release of endorphins, hormones that may reduce the perception of pain.

Studies on people with osteoporosis have confirmed that calcitonin protects bone. However, these studies have only examined short-term use (1 to 2 years), so we don't know how calcitonin works over the long term.[15]

Safety Issues

Until recently, calcitonin had to be taken by injection, but it's now available as a nasal spray. The injected form has caused some minor side effects, including nausea and frequent urination; the only side effect associated with the nasal spray is a runny nose.

But nasal-spray calcitonin is *not* recommended for women within 5 years after menopause, because some evidence indicates that women early into their postmenopausal years may have unpredictable skeletal responses to this therapy.

Tamoxifen

Tamoxifen was developed more than 20 years ago as a birth control pill. Though it didn't work as a contraceptive,

Conventional Treatments for Osteoporosis

it has found widespread use for treating breast cancer. It may be useful against osteoporosis for women who cannot take estrogen because they have had breast cancer. It also improves blood cholesterol levels.

Tamoxifen works in a complex way, apparently having an antiestrogenic effect on breast tissue and a proestrogenic effect on bone. It has been found to significantly increase bone density in the lumbar (lower) spine.[16] However, there isn't much data to say whether tamoxifen actually reduces the incidence of fractures.

Unfortunately, tamoxifen use has a significant downside, too. The most worrisome are statistics that show it increases the risk of uterine cancer by 200 to 300%. Tamoxifen may also increase the risk of liver tumors. The FDA approves the use of tamoxifen, but suggests that women who take it should be monitored closely with regular gynecologic exams.

In addition to these risks, tamoxifen frequently causes side effects, primarily due to its antiestrogenic properties. These include hot flashes, nausea, vaginal irritation, and muscle cramps.

Sodium Fluoride

ERT, calcitonin, and other medications we've discussed protect bone by slowing the rate at which it breaks down. Sodium fluoride works on the other half of the bone remodeling cycle, protecting bone by stimulating the formation of new bone. When combined with calcium supplementation, sodium fluoride holds promise in the treatment of severe osteoporosis. But it has problems, and at present its use is experimental.

High doses of sodium fluoride tend to cause bones to become more crystalline, less elastic, and therefore more brittle than normal bone. Some individuals taking sodium fluoride have experienced side effects of stomach pain, nausea, inflamed joints, and anemia caused by gastrointestinal bleeding. At present, sodium fluoride's potential to increase bone density must be weighed against its risks and side effects. However, new research suggests that specific forms of sodium fluoride, taken intermittently and with calcium supplements, may hold promise as part of an approach to treating osteoporosis.[17]

Evaluation and Screening for Osteoporosis

C ertain groups are at greater risk for osteoporosis than others. But it's hard to say whether you, individually, are at risk. Until recently, there was no way to know for certain until you broke a bone. Today, thanks to advances in medical technology, osteoporosis can be detected earlier, by measuring bone density and the rate of bone loss. This section describes the tests that are currently available to help you assess your own risk for osteoporosis.

Bone Density

The strength and health of a bone can be estimated by measuring the density of the minerals in it. A lower-than-normal bone mineral density (BMD) indicates a greater chance of fracture. Over time, this kind of measurement will also show whether you are gaining or losing bone, and how quickly.

There are a number of techniques for looking at bone density. Basically, they involve either x-ray or ultrasound technology, used in highly specific ways. Tests that can measure bone mineral density include the CT scan, ultrasound, SPA and DPA (single- and dual-photon absorptiometry), and DXA (dual energy x-ray absorptiometry). This last (pronounced "dex-a") test is the one most widely used for assessing an individual's risk for osteoporosis. It exposes people to less radiation than other types of scans (except for ultrasound techniques) and takes less time: 5 to 10 minutes.

The DXA Scan

The DXA scan consists of a special x-ray technique that can assess the density of various bones in the body. Although it is usually used for measuring bone density in the lumbar (lower) spine and the hip, the DXA can also measure bone at the forearm, the finger, the heel, or the whole body.

Normal x rays don't show bone loss until you've lost 30 to 40% of your bone mass. You don't want to wait that long. A DXA scan can identify losses of only 2 to 4%. Thanks to this test, it's possible to detect a dangerous rate of bone loss before it actually causes a fracture. This test, approved in 1988, also has the advantage of taking only a few minutes to perform. With a DXA scan, any area of the body can be measured and a sharper picture can be obtained than with any of the methods previously used.

What About Radiation?

Since the DXA scan uses x-ray technology, it does expose you to a small amount of ionizing radiation. The exposure from a standard DXA (measuring the spine and hip) equals about $\frac{1}{20}$ to $\frac{1}{30}$ the radiation you'd get from a standard two-view chest x-ray. In fact, the DXA scan exposes you to about as much radiation as you'd get sitting in an airplane on a transatlantic flight. (As you may know, cosmic radiation is stronger at the altitudes where planes fly, and passengers as well as crew get exposed to tiny but significant amounts of radiation.)

Of course, it's good to minimize your exposure to radiation, but the amount you'd get from a DXA scan shouldn't be a concern.

What Does a DXA Scan Tell You?

When you get a DXA scan, you find out how your bone mineral density compares with two averages. Multiple DXA scans over time can also tell you at what rate you're losing bone.

Your DXA scan results will include two scores. One compares your BMD to that of an average, healthy young adult of your sex. The other compares your results with those of an average, healthy adult your own age. As you might guess, the lower these scores, the greater your risk for fracturing a bone in the near future.

Postmenopausal women may lose between 1 and 5% of their bone mass each year. By getting repeat DXA scans every 2 years, you can learn how quickly you're losing bone. If you are a "fast loser," meaning that you are losing 3% or more each year, you definitely need to take charge of the situation. In consultation with your physician, choose a plan of action and stick to it. Follow-up DXA scans, and possibly some of the bone markers discussed in the following sections, will show you how well the treatment is working.

A Promising Method to Measure the Rate of Bone Loss

Other tests measure the chemicals in the urine that are produced in the process of bone resorption. Measuring these "bone breakdown products," according to some

What Do Your DXA Scan Results Mean?

If you have a DXA scan, your health-care provider will use two scores to evaluate your results: A "T score," which compares your bone mineral density against an average healthy young adult's; and a "Z score," which shows where you stand in your own age group. Your health-care provider will recommend treatment based on which category your scores place you in.

For example, if your T score shows that your bone mineral density is close to an average young adult's, you're in good shape. If you are near menopause or have already entered it, your health-care provider may request that you repeat the test in 5 years.

If your T score is slightly below zero (meaning that your bone mineral density is a bit lower than a young adult's), but

experts, may be a promising way to diagnose osteoporosis even sooner than a DXA scan can. The hope is that these urine tests can show the rate of bone loss in a single test. As we've seen, you can't get the rate of bone loss with only a single DXA scan; you have to take multiple scans every 16 months to learn how quickly you're losing bone.

Another possible advantage to these urine tests is that they're less expensive than a DXA scan. The cost of a DXA scan can be the deciding factor for some people.

The urine tests (including tests called Pyrilinks, Pyrilinks-D, and Osteomark-NTX) measure bone breakdown products, and therefore give an indication of how quickly bone is being resorbed.

However, these tests can't tell you exactly what your bone mineral density is at the present, and their exact use-your Z score is normal for your age, you have evidence of bone loss, but not more than the average person your age. Your health-care provider may request that you repeat the test in 2 to 3 years.

If your T score is somewhat lower—between -2.0 and -2.5—your health care provider may tell you that you have "osteopenia," a precursor to osteoporosis, and may suggest treatment.

If both your T scores and Z scores are low, with your T score falling below -2.5, you have osteoporosis. You might have a fracture that shows up on the scan, or you might have already broken a bone. Your physician will offer you a treatment program.[1]

fulness hasn't been completely determined yet. For more information about these tests, consult your health-care provider.

When Should You Get Your Bone Mineral Density Tested?

Most health-care plans will reimburse you for a DXA scan if you're at high risk for osteoporosis. To be specific, your health insurer will probably cover the cost of a DXA scan if you have a history of a non-impact (spontaneous) fracture as an adult, if you're considered at high risk for bone loss (see chapter 2 for the recognized risk factors), or if you're a menopausal woman who is not on hormone replacement therapy.

Meredith's Story

Meredith, a university professor in her mid 50s, went to her doctor's office with a fractured wrist. While playing golf, she'd tripped and fallen. Even though the injury had happened some time ago and her cast had been removed, Meredith's wrist wasn't completely healed.

After recommending some treatments to help her bones heal more quickly, Meredith's doctor suggested that she get a DXA scan of her hip and spine, to see if her wrist fracture was simply the result of a bad fall, or whether she had osteoporosis and her wrist was unusually weak. The results of her DXA scan revealed that her T score (the comparison with the bone of

Some experts believe that women at high risk should have a DXA scan even at 20 and 30 years of age, while all women should have a test at age 40 to determine a baseline for future reference. This type of intensive monitoring may not be available to everyone, and a DXA scan can cost anywhere from $150.00 in a research setting to $250.00 or more through a radiology laboratory or local hospital. However, organizations within your community may offer free or reduced bone mineral density scans at certain times of the year. Keep alert to community or hospital health fairs, public health announcements, or the activities of women's health organizations.

Whether or not you use these tests, it makes sense to start with some preventive measures. Many of the natural treatments and diet, exercise, and lifestyle changes recommended here can be safely used by any healthy adult as young women in their 20s) was -2.3, showing that Meredith was indeed losing bone and that her risk for fracture was more than four times higher than that of someone without bone loss. Because she was not taking estrogen (she had opted out due to a history of gallbladder problems), her doctor suggested that she start resistance training 3 times weekly, take calcium and a mineral supplement, and take ipriflavone. Over the next 4 years her DXA scan improved so much that she was no longer "osteopenic" (bone loss that is measurable but not bad enough to be considered osteoporosis).

prevention. If you're concerned about osteoporosis but a DXA scan isn't within your means, you can still discuss your concerns with your health care provider and choose an approach that fits you.

Putting It All Together

O f Americans over age 50, 20% of women and 5% of men have osteoporosis. This serious disease causes the bones to become progressively lighter and weaker until they are dangerously easy to break, especially in the hips, spine, and wrists. Though some groups of people have a higher risk, men and women of all ages and races get osteoporosis.

Conventional Therapies

The leading conventional therapy to prevent menopause-related osteoporosis is estrogen, taken either by itself as estrogen replacement therapy (ERT) or in combination with a progestin as hormone replacement therapy (HRT). Taking estrogen after menopause protects woman against bone loss and reduces the risk of a fracture by about 50%. But estrogen comes with side effects and health risks, and many women cannot or choose not to take it.

Medical research is working on medications that can provide estrogen's health benefits without its risks and side effects. One such drug has been recently approved for use: raloxifene (Evista). Other effective conventional treatments for osteoporosis include calcitonin and alendronate (Fosamax).

Calcium and Vitamin D

Calcium and vitamin D play important roles in forming and protecting bone. Research shows that calcium supplements, especially when combined with vitamin D supplements, can significantly protect against bone loss. There is also evidence that using calcium and vitamin D supplements can increase the effectiveness of HRT, allowing you to get bone-protecting benefit from a low dosage of estrogen.

The best-absorbed form of calcium appears to be a chelated supplement (for example, calcium citrate or calcium citrate malate). Adults (other than pregnant women) should have a total calcium intake of about 1,000 to 1,500 mg daily (refer to table 2 for more specific dosage information). The usual recommended dosage for vitamin D is 400 to 800 IU daily.

Ipriflavone

Closely related to substances found in soybeans, ipriflavone has been extensively studied and found to be effective in protecting and building bone mass in postmenopausal women.

Ipriflavone seems to be about as effective as estrogen replacement therapy for osteoporosis. The apparent advantage of ipriflavone is that it has virtually no side effects, and appears to be without any significant health risks. However, it does not reduce symptoms of menopause and may not offer some of the other health benefits of estrogen. The usual dosage for ipriflavone is 600 mg daily.

Helpful Vitamins and Minerals

Vitamin K plays a role in bone formation, and recent evidence indicates that including more of it in your diet might help protect you against osteoporosis. Vitamin K is found in lettuce and other green, leafy vegetables.

Other vitamins and minerals that may play a helpful role in protecting bone include magnesium, vitamin B_6, manganese, boron, zinc, copper, and silicon.

Lifestyle Issues

Exercise is one of the most important ways to fight osteoporosis. Vigorous weight-bearing exercise can protect and even build bone mass.

Too much sodium and phosphorus in your diet can cause you to lose calcium. By guarding against excessive intakes of both, you can effectively increase your body's ability to benefit from the calcium in your diet.

New evidence has made it hard to say for certain whether a high-protein diet hurts or helps your bones.

Progesterone

Progesterone and its chemical cousins, the progestins, are used to help reduce the risk of uterine cancer associated with taking estrogen. While there is preliminary evidence that progesterone may be beneficial in preventing and reducing osteoporosis by increasing bone formation, one well-designed study found no improvement in bone mass in postmenopausal women using progesterone cream topically.

Detecting Osteoporosis

The best way to measure your personal risk for osteoporosis is the DXA scan. This safe test can tell you your bone mineral density. When repeated over time, bone scans can also show whether you're losing bone.

Notes

Chapter 1
What Is Osteoporosis?

1. Lane NE. *The Osteoporosis Book: A Guide for Patients and Their Families.* New York: Oxford University Press; 1999:xiii.

2. Lonzer D, Imrie R, Rogers D, et al. Effects of heredity, age, weight, puberty, activity, and calcium intake on bone mineral density in children. *Clin Pediatr.* 1996;35:185–189.

3. Osteoporosis and Related Bone Diseases National Resource Center. Gallup survey on National Osteoporosis Foundation. Dr. Eric Orwoll of Portland Veterans Administration Medical Center cites figures: 1.5 million men have osteoporosis, 3.5 million are at risk.

4. Lane NE. *The Osteoporosis Book: A Guide for Patients and Their Families.* New York: Oxford University Press; 1999:9.

5. Scheiber LB II, Torregrosa L. Evaluation and treatment of postmenopausal osteoporosis. *Semin Arthritis Rheum.* 1998;27:245-261.

6. Lane NE. *The Osteoporosis Book: A Guide for Patients and Their Families.* New York: Oxford University Press; 1999:12–13.

7. Lane NE. *The Osteoporosis Book: A Guide for Patients and Their Families.* New York: Oxford University Press; 1999:13–15.

8. Osteoporosis and Related Bone Diseases National Resource Center. A program sponsored by the NIH Institute of Arthritis and Musculoskeletal and Skin Diseases.

9. Lane NE. *The Osteoporosis Book: A Guide for Patients and Their Families.* New York: Oxford University Press; 1999:3.

10. Cummings SR, Black DM, Rubin SM. Lifetime risks of hip, Colles', or vertebral fracture and coronary heart disease among white postmenopausal women. *Arch Intern Med.* 1989;149:2445–2448.

11. Lane NE. *The Osteoporosis Book: A Guide for Patients and Their Families.* New York: Oxford University Press; 1999:3–5.

12. Lees B, Molleson T, Arnett T, et al. Differences in proximal femur bone density over two centuries. *Lancet.* 1993;341:673–675.

13. Wallace WA. The increasing incidence of fractures of the proximal femur: An orthopaedic epidemic. *Lancet.* 1983;1:1413–1414.

14. Boyce WJ, Vessey MP. Rising incidence of fracture of the proximal femur. *Lancet.* 1985;1:150–151.

15. Johnell O, Nilsson B, Obrant K, et al. Age and sex patterns of hip fracture changes in 30 years. *Acta Orthop Scand.* 1984;55:290–292.

Chapter 2
Who Is at Risk?

1. Seeman E. Advances in the study of osteoporosis in men. In: Meunier PJ, ed. *Osteoporosis: Diagnosis and Management.* St. Louis: Mosby; 1998:211.

2. Bonnick SL. *The Osteoporosis Handbook.* New York: Taylor Publishing Company; 1994:20–21.

3. Johnell O, Gullberg B, Kanis JA, et al. Risk factors for hip fracture in European women: the MEDOS study. Mediterranean Osteoporosis Study. *J Bone Miner Res.* 1995;10:1802–1815.

4. Yurth EF. Female athlete triad. *West J Med.* 1995;162:149–150.

5. Maggi S, Kelsey JL, Litvak J, et al. Incidence of hip fractures in the elderly: a cross-national analysis. *Osteoporos Int.* 1991;1:232–241.

6. Arden N, Cooper C. Present and future of osteoporosis: epidemiology. In Meunier PJ, ed. *Osteoporosis: Diagnosis and Management.* St. Louis: Mosby; 1998:1–17.

7. Slemenda CW, Hui SL, Longscope C, et al. Predictors of bone mass in perimenopausal women: a prospective study of clinical data using photon absorbtiometry. *Ann Intern Med.* 1990;112:96–101.

8. Matkovic V, Fontana D, Tominac C, et al. Factors that influence peak bone mass formation: a study of calcium balance and the inheritance of bone mass in adolescent females. *Am J Clin Nutr.* 1990;52:878–888.

9. Johnston C, Miller J, Slemenda C, et al. Calcium supplementation and increases in bone mineral density in children. *N Engl J Med.* 1992;327:82–87.

10. Slemenda CW, Miller J, Hui S, et al. Role of physical activity in the development of skeletal mass in children. *J Bone Miner Res.* 1991;6:1227–1233.

11. Lane NE. *The Osteoporosis Book: A Guide for Patients and Their Families.* New York: Oxford University Press; 1999:21–22.

12. Lane NE. *The Osteoporosis Book: A Guide for Patients and Their Families.* New York: Oxford University Press; 1999:16–17.

13. Kanis JA. *Textbook of Osteoporosis.* England: Blackwell Science Ltd.; 1996:164.

14. Toogood JH. Side effects of inhaled corticosteriods. *J Allergy Clin Immunol.* 1998;102:705–713.

15. Medical Economics. *Physicians Desk Reference.* Montvale, NJ: Medical Economics Company; 1999:2472.

16. Cundy T, Evans M, Roberts H, et al. Bone density in women receiving depot medroxyprogesterone acetate for contraception. *Br Med J.* 1991;303:13–16.

17. Cundy T. Recovery of bone density in women who stop using medroxyprogesterone acetate. *Br Med J.* 1994;308:247–248.

18. Johansen JS, Riis BJ, Hassager C, et al. The effect of a gonadotropin-releasing hormone analog (nafarelin) on bone metabolism. *J Clin Endocrinol Metab.* 1988;67:701–706.

19. Bonnick SL. *The Osteoporosis Handbook.* Texas: Taylor Publishing Company; 1994:20–21.

20. Kanis JA. *Textbook of Osteoporosis.* England: Blackwell Science Ltd.; 1996:164.

21. Schnitzler CM, Solomon L. Bone changes after alcohol abuse. *S Afr Med J.* 1984;66:730–734.

22. Crilly RG, Anderson C, Hogan D, et al. Bone histomorphometry, bone mass, and related parameters in alcoholic males. *Calcif Tissue Int.* 1988;43:269–276.

23. Hansen MA, Overgaard K, Riis BJ, et al. Potential risk factors for development of postmenopausal osteoporosis–examined over a 12-year period. *Osteoporos Int.* 1991;1:95–102.

24. Holbrook TL, Barrett-Connor E. A prospective study of alcohol consumption and bone mineral density. *Br Med J.* 1993;306:1506–1509.

25. Kimble RB. Alcohol, cytokines, and estrogen in the control of bone remodeling. *Alcohol Clin Exp Res.* 1997;21:385–391.

26 Slemenda CW. Adult Bone Loss. In: Marcus R, ed. *Osteoporosis.* Boston: Blackwell Science Inc.; 1994:107–124.

27. Law M. Smoking and Osteoporosis. In: Wald W, Baron J, eds. *Smoking and Hormone-Related Disorders.* Oxford: Oxford Medical Publications; 1990.

28. Daniell H. Osteoporosis of the slender smoker. *Arch Intern Med.* 1976;136:298–304.

29. Krall EA, Dawson-Hughes B. Smoking and bone loss among post-menopausal women. *J Bone Miner Res.* 1991;6:331–338.

30. Slemenda CW, Christian JC, Reed T, et al. Long-term bone loss in men: effects of genetic and environmental factors. *Annals Intern Med.* 1992;117:286-291.

31. Kerstetter JE, Allen LH. Protein intake and calcium homeostasis. *Adv Nutr Res.* 1994;9:167–181.

32. Heaney RP, Gallagher JC, Johnston CC, et al. Calcium nutrition and bone health in the elderly. *Am J Clin Nutr.* 1982;36:986–1013.

33. Heaney R. Excess dietary protein may not adversely affect bone. *J Nutr.* 1998;128:1054–1057.

34. Munger R, Cerhan J, Chiu B. Prospective study of dietary protein intake and risk of hip fracture in postmenopausal women. *Am J Clin Nutr.* 1999;69:147–152.

35. Devine A, Criddle RA, Dick IM, et al. A longitudinal study of the effect of sodium and calcium intakes on regional bone density in postmenopausal women. *Am J Clin Nutr.* 1995;62:740–745.

36. Massey LK, Whiting SJ. Dietary salt, urinary calcium, and bone loss. *J Bone Miner Res.* 1996;11:731–736.

37. Heaney RP, Recker RR. Effects of nitrogen, phosphorus, and caffeine on calcium balance in women. *J Lab Clin Med.* 1982;99:46–55.

38. Kiel DP, Felson DT, Hannan MT, et al. Caffeine and the risk of hip fracture: the Framingham study. *Am J Epidemiol.* 1990;132:675–684.

39. Johnell O, Gullberg B, Kanis JA, et al. Risk factors for hip fracture in European women: the MEDOS study. Mediterranean Osteoporosis Study. *J Bone Miner Res.* 1995;10:1802–1815.

Chapter 3
Menopause, Estrogen, and Osteoporosis

1. Stevenson J, et al. Determinants of bone density in normal women: Risk factors for future osteoporosis. *Br Med J.* 1989;298:924–928.

2. Delmas PD. Hormone replacement therapy in the prevention and treatment of osteoporosis. *Osteoporos Int.* 1997;7(suppl 1):S3–S7.

3. Ettinger B. Postmenopausal Osteoporosis. *Curr Ther Endocrinol Metab.* 1997;6:639–644.

4. Johnell O, Gullberg B, Kanis JA, et al. Risk factors for hip fracture in European women: the MEDOS study. Mediterranean Osteoporosis Study. *J Bone Miner Res.* 1995;10:1802–1815.

5. Yurth EF. Female athlete triad. *West J Med.* 1995;162:149–150.

6. Kadel NJ, Teitz CC, Kronmal RA. Stress fractures in ballet dancers. *Am J Sports Med.* 1992;20:445–449.

7. Yurth EF. Female athlete triad. *West J Med.* 1995;162:149–150.

8. Rigotti NA, Neer RM, Skates SJ, et al. The clinical course of osteoporosis in anorexia nervosa: a longitudinal study of cortical bone mass. *JAMA.* 1991;265:1133–1138.

9. Delmas PD. Hormone replacement therapy in the prevention and treatment of osteoporosis. *Osteoporos Int.* 1997;7(suppl 1):S3–S7.

10. Genant HK, Baylink DJ, Gallagher JC. Estrogens in the prevention of osteoporosis in postmenopausal women. *Am J Obstet Gynecol.* 1989;161:1842–1846.

11. Ross RK, Paganini-Hill A, Wan PC, et al. Effect of hormone replacement therapy on breast cancer risk: estrogen versus estrogen plus progestin. *J Natl Cancer Inst.* 2000;92:328–332.

12. Schairer C, Lubin J, Troisi R, et al. Menopausal estrogen and estrogen-progestin replacement therapy and breast cancer risk. *JAMA.* 2000;283:485–491.

13. Nozaki M, Hashimoto K, Inoue Y, et al. Treatment of bone loss in oophorectomized women with a combination of ipriflavone and conjugated equine estrogen. *Int J Gynecol Obstet.* 1998;62:69–75.

14. Melis GB, Paoletti AM, Bartolini R, et al. Ipriflavone and low doses of estrogens in the prevention of bone mineral loss in climacterium. *Bone Miner.* 1992;19(suppl):S49–S56.

15. Yamazaki I, Shino A, Shimizu Y, et al. Effect of ipriflavone on glucocorticoid-induced osteoporosis in rats. *Life Sci.* 1986;38:951–958.

Chapter 4
Calcium and Vitamin D for Osteoporosis

1. Eaton SB, Konner M. Paleolithic nutrition: a consideration of its nature and current implications. *N Engl J Med.* 1985;312:283–289.

2. Heaney RP. Non-pharmacologic prevention of osteoporosis: nutrition and exercise. In: Meunier PJ, ed. *Osteoporosis: Diagnosis and Management.* St. Louis: Mosby; 1998:162–163.

3. U.S. Department of Agriculture, Agricultural Research Service. 1997. Data tables: Results from USDA's 1994–96 Continuing Survey of Food Intakes by Individuals and 1994–96 Diet and Health Knowledge Survey. On: 1994–96 Continuing Survey of Food Intakes by Individuals and 1994–96 Diet and Health Knowledge Survey. CD-ROM, NTIS Accession Number PB98–500457.

4. Gebhardt S, Matthews R. *Nutritive Values of Foods.* USDA; 1981.

5. Pennington J and Church H. *Food Values of Portions Commonly Used.* New York: Harper and Row; 1985.

6. Brown S. *Better Bones Better Body.* New Caanan: Keats Publishing; 1996.

7. Bachrach L. Bone acquisition in childhood and adolescence. In: Marcus R, ed. *Osteoporosis.* Boston; Blackwell Science Inc.; 1994:49–68.

8. Lloyd T, Andon MB, Rollings N, et al. Calcium supplementation and bone mineral density in adolescent girls. *JAMA.* 1993;270:841–844.

9. Matkovic V, Kostial K, Simonovic I, et al. Bone status and fracture rates in two regions of Yugoslavia. *Am J Clin Nutr.* 1979;32:540–549.

10. Matkovic V, Fontana D, Tominac C, et. al. Factors that influence peak bone mass formation: a study of calcium balance and the inheritance of bone mass in adolescent females. *Am J Clin Nutr.* 1990;52:878–888.

11. Lloyd T, Andon MB, Rollings N. Calcium supplementation and bone mineral density in adolescent girls. *J Am Med Assoc.* 1993;270:841–844.

12. Lloyd T, Martel JK, Rollings N. The effect of calcium supplementation and Tanner stage on bone density, content and area in teenage women. *Osteoporos Int.* 1996;6:276–283.

13. Johnston C, Miller J, Slemenda C, et al. Calcium supplementation and increases in bone mineral density in children. *N Engl J Med.* 1992;327:82–87.

14. Cumming RG. Calcium intake and bone mass: a quantitative review of the evidence. *Calcif Tissue Int.* 1990;47:194–201.

15. Dawson-Hughes B, Dallal GE, Krall EA, et al. A controlled trial of the effect of calcium supplementation on bone density in postmenopausal women. *N Engl J Med.* 1990;323:870–883.

16. Reid IR, Ames RW, Evans MC, et al. Long-term effects of calcium supplementation on bone loss and fractures in postmenopausal women: a randomized controlled trial. *Am J Med.* 1995;98:331–335.

17. Feskanich D, Willett WC, Stampfer MJ, et al. Milk, dietary calcium, and bone fractures in women: a 12-year prospective study. *Am J Public Health.* 1997;87:992–997.

18. Shearer MJ. The roles of vitamins D and K in bone health and osteoporosis prevention. *Proc Nutr Soc.* 1997;56:915–937.

19. Utiger RD. The need for more vitamin D. *N Engl J Med.* 1998;338:828–829.

20. Prince R. Diet and the prevention of osteoporotic fractures. *N Eng J Med.* 1997;337:701–702.

21. Dawson-Hughes B, Dallal GE, Krall EA, et al. Effect of vitamin D supplementation on wintertime and overall bone loss in healthy postmenopausal women. *Ann Intern Med.* 1991;115:505–512.

22. Dawson-Hughes B, Harris S, Krall E, et al. Effect of calcium and vitamin D supplementation on bone density in men and women 65 years of age or older. *N Eng J Med.* 1997;337:670–673.

23. Chapuy M, Meunier P. Prevention of secondary hyperparathyroidism and hip fracture in elderly women with calcium and vitamin D_3 supplements. *Osteoporos Int.* 1996;6:60–63.

24. Nieves JW, Komar L, Cosman F, et al. Calcium potentiates the effect of estrogen and calcitonin on bone mass: review and analysis. *Am J Clin Nutr.* 1998;67:18–24.

25. Recker RR, Davies KM, Dowd RM, et al. The effect of low-dose continuous estrogen and progesterone therapy with calcium and vitamin D on bone in elderly women: A randomized, controlled trial. *Ann Intern Med.* 1999;130:897–904.

26. Reid IR, Ibbertson HK. Calcium supplements in the prevention of steroid-induced osteoporosis. *Am J Clin Nutr.* 1986;44:287–290.

27. Buckley LM, Leib ES, Cartularo KS, et al. Calcium and vitamin D supplementation prevents bone loss in the spine secondary to low-dose corticosteroids in patients with rheumatoid arthritis. A randomized, double-blind placebo-controlled trial. *Ann Intern Med.* 1996;125:961–68.

28. Norman AW. *Vitamin D: The Calcium Homeostatic Steroid Hormone.* New York: Academic Press; 1979.

29. Stamp TCB, Round JM, Rowe DJF, et al. Plasma levels and therapeutic effects of 25-hydroxy-cholecalciferol in epileptic patients taking anticonvulsant drugs. *Br Med J.* 1972;4:9–12.

30. Holmes T, Kummerow F. The relationship of adequate and excesive intake of vitamin D to health and disease. *J Am Coll Nutr.* 1983;2:173-99.

31. Bourgoin B, Evans D, Cornett JR, et al. Lead content in 70 brands of dietary calcium supplements. *Am J Public Health.* 1993;83:1155–1160.

32. Brennan MJ, Duncan WE, Wartofsky L, et al. In vitro dissolution of calcium carbonate preparations. *Calcif Tissue Int.* 1991;49:308–312.

33. Sheikh MS, Santa Ana CA, Nicar MJ, et al. Gastrointestinal absorption of calcium from milk and calcium salts. *N Engl J Med.* 1987;317:532–536.

34. Dawson-Hughes B, Dallal GE, Krall EA, et al. A controlled trial of the effect of calcium supplementation on bone density in postmenopausal women. *N Engl J Med.* 1990;323:870–883.

35. Khashayar Sakhaee MD. Presented at the American Society for Bone and Mineral Research and the International Bone and Mineral Society; Center for Mineral Metabolism and Clinical Research; Dallas, Texas.

36. Miller J, Smith DL, Flora L, et al. Calcium absorption from calcium carbonate and a new form of calcium (CCM) in healthy male and female adolescents. *Am J Clin Nutr.* 1988;48:1291–1294.

37. Utiger RD. The need for more vitamin D. *N Engl J Med.* 1998;338:828–829.

38. National Institutes of Health. *Consensus Development Panel on Optimal Calcium Intake.* National Institutes of Health; 1994.

39. Curhan GC, Willett WC, Rimm EB. A prospective study of dietary calcium and supplemental calcium and other nutrients as factors affecting the risk of kidney stones in women. *Ann Int Med.* 1997:126:497–504.

40. Curhan GC, Willett WC, Rimm EB, et al. A prospective study of dietary calcium and other nutrients and the risk of symptomatic kidney stones. *N Engl J Med.* 1993;l328:833–838.

41. Argiratos V, Samman S. The effect of calcium carbonate and calcium citrate on the absorption of zinc in healthy female subjects. *Eur J Clin Nutr.* 1994;48:198–204.

42. Hwang SJ, Lai YH, Chen HC, et al. Comparisons of the effects of calcium carbonate and calcium acetate on zinc tolerance test in hemodialysis patients. *Am J Kidney Dis.* 1992;19:57–60.

43. Pecoud A, Donzel P, Schelling JL. Effect of foodstuffs on the absorption of zinc sulfate. *Clin Pharmacol Ther.* 1975;17:469–474.

44. Spencer H, Kramer L, Norris C, et al. Effect of calcium and phosphorus on zinc metabolism in man. *Am J Clin Nutr.* 1984;40:1213–1218.

45. Dawson-Hughes B, Seligson FH, Hughes VA. Effects of calcium carbonate and hydroxyapatite on zinc and iron retention in postmenopausal women. *Am J Clin Nutr.* 1986;44:83–88.

46. Seaborn C, Stoecker B. Effect of antacid or ascorbic acid on tissue accumulation and urinary excretion of chromium. *Nutr Res.* 1990;10:1401–1407.

47. Hallberg L, Brune M, Erlandsson M, et al. Calcium: effect of different amounts on nonheme- and heme-iron absorption in humans. *Am J Clin Nutr.* 1991;53:112–119.

48. Cook JD, Dassenko SA, Whittaker P. Calcium supplementation: effect on iron absorption. *Am J Clin Nutr.* 1991;53:106–111.

49. Freeland-Graves JH, Lin PH. Plasma uptake of manganese as affected by oral loads of manganese, calcium, milk, phosphorus, copper and zinc. *J Am Coll Nutr.* 1991;10:38–43.

50. Davidsson L, Cederblad A, Lonnerdal B, et al. The effect of individual dietary components on manganese absorption in humans. *Am J Clin Nutr.* 1991;54:1065–1070.

51. Carter BL, Garnett WR, Pellock JM, et al. Effect of antacids on phenytoin bioavailability. *Ther Drug Monit.* 1981;3:333–340.

52. McElnay JC, Uprichard G, Collier PS. The effect of activated dimethicone and a proprietary antacid preparation containing this agent on the absorption of phenytoin. *Br J Clin Pharmacol.* 1982;13:501–505.

53. Wahl TO, Gobuty AH, Lukert BP. Long-term anticonvulsant therapy and intestinal calcium absorption. *Clin Pharmacol Ther.* 1981;30:506–512.

54. Weinstein RS, Bryce GF, Sappington LJ, et al. Decreased serum ionized calcium and normal vitamin D metabolite levels with anticonvulsant drug treatment. *J Clin Endocrinol Metab.* 1984;58:1003–1009.

55. Hahn TJ, Hendin BA, Scharp CR, et al. Effect of chronic anticonvulsant therapy on serum 25-hydroxycalciferol levels in adults. *N Engl J Med.* 1972;287:900–904.

56. Jubiz W, Haussler MR, McCain TA, et al. Plasma 1,25-dihydroxyvitamin D levels in patients receiving anticonvulsant drugs. *J Clin Endocrinol Metab.* 1977;44:617–621.

57. Williams C, Netzloff M, Folkerts L, et al. Vitamin D metabolism and anticonvulsant therapy: effect of sunshine on incidence of osteomalacia. *South Med J.* 1984;77:834–836, 842.

58. Tomita S, Ohnishi J, Nakano M, et al. The effects of anticonvulsant drugs on vitamin D_3-activating cytochrome P-450-linked monooxygenase systems. *J Steroid Biochem Mol Biol.* 1991;39:479–485.

59. Weinstein RS, Bryce GF, Sappington LJ, et al. Decreased serum ionized calcium and normal vitamin D metabolite levels with anticonvulsant drug treatment. *J Clin Endocrinol Metab.* 1984;58:1003–1009.

60. Buckley LM, Leib ES, Cartularo KS, et al. Calcium and vitamin D_3 supplementation prevents bone loss in the spine secondary to low-dose corticosteroids in patients with rheumatoid arthritis. A randomized, double-blind, placebo-controlled trial. *Ann Intern Med.* 1996;125:961 68.

61. Reid IR, Ibbertson HK. Calcium supplements in the prevention of steroid-induced osteoporosis. *Am J Clin Nutr.* 1986;44:287–90

62. Neuvonen PJ. Interactions with the absorption of tetracyclines. *Drugs.* 1976;11:45–54.

63. Neuvonen PJ, Kivisto KT, Lehto P. Interference of dairy products with the absorption of ciprofloxacin. *Clin Pharmacol Ther.* 1991;50:498–502.

64. Minami R, Inotsume N, Nakano M, et al. Effect of milk on absorption of norfloxacin in healthy volunteers. *J Clin Pharmacol.* 1993;33:1238–1240.

65. Kirch W, Schafer-Korting M, Axthelm T, et al. Interaction of atenolol with furosemide and calcium and aluminum salts. *Clin Pharmacol Ther.* 1981;4:429–435.

66. Kuhn M, Schriger DL. Low-dose calcium pretreatment to prevent verapamil-induced hypotension. *Am Heart J.* 1992;124:231–32.

67. David BO, et al. Calcium and calciferol antagonize effect of verapamil in atrial fibrillation. *Br Med J.* 1981;282:1585–1586.

68. Hariman RJ, Mangiardi LM, McAllister RG Jr, et al. Reversal of the cardiovascular effects of verapamil by calcium and sodium: differences between electrophysiologic and hemodynamic responses. *Circulation.* 1979;59:797–804.

69. Watanabe Y, Nishimura M. Calcium–verapamil interaction on the AV node. *Int J Cardiol.* 1984;6:275–276.

70. Guadagnino V, Greengart A, Hollander G, et al. Treatment of severe left ventricular dysfunction with calcium chloride in patients receiving verapamil. *J Clin Pharmacol.* 1987;27:407–409.

71. Salerno DM, Anderson B Sharkey PJ, et al. Intravenous verapamil for treatment of multifocal atrial tachycardia with and without calcium pretreatment. *Ann Intern Med.* 1987;107:623–628.

72. Riis B, Christiansen C. Actions of thiazide on vitamin D metabolism: a controlled therapeutic trial in normal women early in the postmenopause. *Metabolism.* 1985;34:421–24.

73. Lemann J Jr, Gray RW, Maierhofer WJ, et al. Hydrochlorothiazide inhibits bone resorption in men despite experimentally elevated serum 1,25-dihydroxyvitamin D concentrations. *Kidney Int.* 1985;28:951–958.

74. Crowe M, Wollner L, Griffiths RA. Hypercalcaemia following vitamin D and thiazide therapy in the elderly. *Practitioner.* 1984;228:312–313.

75. Gora ML, Seth SK, Bay WH, et al. Milk-alkali syndrome associated with use of chlorothiazide and calcium carbonate. *Clin Pharm.* 1989;8:227–229.

76. Kupfer S, Kosovsky JD. Effects of cardiac glycosides on renal tubular transport of calcium, magnesium, inorganic phosphate and glucose in the dog. *J Clin Invest.* 1965;44:1132–43.

77. Nolan CR, Califano JR, Butzin CA. Influence of calcium acetate or calcium citrate on intestinal aluminum absorption. *Kidney Int.* 1990;38:937–941.

78. [No author listed]. Preliminary findings suggest calcium citrate supplements may raise aluminum levels in blood, urine. *Fam Pract News.* 1992;22:74–75.

79. Odes HS. Effect of cimetidine on hepatic vitamin D metabolism in humans. *Digestion.* 1990;46:61–64.

80. Bengoa JM, Bolt MJ, Rosenberg IH. Hepatic vitamin D 25-hydroxylase inhibition by cimetidine and isonizid. *J Lab Clin Med.* 1984;104:546–552.

81. Bengoa JM. Cimetidine inhibits the hepatic hydroxylation of vitamin D. *Nutr Rev.* 1985;43:184–185.

82. Aarskog D, Aksens L, Markestad TK, et al. Heparin induced inhibition of 1,25-dihydroxyvitamin D formation. *Am J Obstet Gynecol.* 1984;148:1141–1142.

83. Haram K, Hervig T, Thordarson H, et al. Osteopenia caused by heparin treatment in pregnancy. *Acta Obstet Gynecol Scand.* 1993;72:674–675.

84. Wise PH, Hall AS. Heparin induced osteopenia in pregnancy. *Br Med J.* 1980;281:110–111.

85. Perry W, Erooga MA, Brown J, et al. Calcium metabolism during rifampicin and isoniazid therapy for tuberculosis. *J R Soc Med.* 1982;75:533–536.

86. Brodie MJ, Boobis AR, Hillyard CJ, et al. Effect of isoniazid on vitamin D metabolism and hepatic monooxygenase activity. *Clin Pharmacol Ther.* 1981;30:363–7.

Chapter 5
Ipriflavone and Phytoestrogens

1. Anderson JW, Johnstone BM, Cook-Newell ME. Meta-analysis of effects of soy protein on serum lipids. *N Engl J Med.* 1995;333:276–282.

2. Messina MJ, Persky V, Setchell KD, et al. Soy intake and cancer risk: a review of the *in vitro* and *in vivo* data. *Nutr Cancer.* 1994;21:113–131.

3. Messina M, Messina V. Soyfoods, soybean isoflavones, and bone health: a brief overview. *J Ren Nutr.* 2000;10:63–68.

4. Cassidy A, Bingham S, Setchell K. Biological effects of a diet of soy protein rich in isoflavones on the menstrual cycle of pre-menopausal women. *Am J Clin Nutr.* 1994;60:333–340.

5. Anderson J. *Isoflavone concentration in soyfoods.* Presented at: American Dietetics Association's 80th Annual Meeting. October 27–30, 1997; Boston, Mass.

6. Anderson JB, Ambrose WW, Garner SC. Biphasic effects of genistein on bone tissue in the ovariectomized, lactating rat model. *Proc Soc Exp Biol Med.* 1998;217:345–350.

7. Potter SM, Baum JA, Teng H, et al. Soy protein and isoflavones: their effects on blood lipids and bone density in postmenopausal women. *Am J Clin Nutr.* 1998;68(suppl);S1375–S1379.

8. Nagata C, Kabuto M, Kurisu Y, et al. Decreased serum estra-diol concentration associated with high dietary intake of soy products in premenopausal Japanese women. *Nutr Cancer.* 1997;29:228–233.

9. Lee HP, Gourley L, Duffy SW, et al. Dietary effects on breast-cancer risk in Singapore. *Lancet.* 1991;337:1197–1200.

10. Ingram D, Sanders K, Kolybaba M, et al. Case-control study of phyto-oestrogens and breast cancer. *Lancet.* 1997;350:990–994.

11. McMichael-Phillips DF, Harding C, Morton M, et al. Effects of soy-protein supplementation on epithelial proliferation in the histologically normal human breast. *Am J Clin Nutr.* 1998;68(suppl 6):S1431–S1435.

12. Anderson J, Murkies A, Lombard C. Dietary flour supplemen-tation decreases postmenopausal hot flushes: effect of soy and wheat. Second International Symposium on the Role of Soy in Preventing and Treating Chronic Disease; September 15-18, 1996; Brussels, Belgium.

13. Potter SM, Baum JA, Teng H, et al. Soy protein and isoflavones: their effects on blood lipids and bone density in postmenopausal women. *Am J Clin Nutr.* 1998;68(suppl):S1375–S1379.

14. Brandi ML. New treatment strategies: ipriflavone, strontium, vitamin D metabolites and analogs. *Am J Med.* 1993;95(suppl 5A):69S–74S.

15. Melis G, Paoletti A, Cagnacci A, et al. Lack of any estrogenic effect of ipriflavone in postmenopausal women. *J Endocrinol Invest.* 1992;15:755–761.

16. Petilli M, Fiorelli G, Benvenuti U, et al. Interactions between ipriflavone and the estrogen receptor. *Calcif Tissue Int.* 1995;156:160–165.

17. Civitelli R. *In vitro* and *in vivo* effects of ipriflavone on bone formation and bone biomechanics. *Calcif Tissue Int.* 1997;61:S12–S14.

18. Cheng SL, Zhang TL, Nelson TL, et al. Stimulation of human osteoblast differentiation and function by ipriflavone and its metabolites. *Calcif Tissue Int.* 1994;55:356–362.

19. Civitelli R. *In vitro* and *in vivo* effects of ipriflavone on bone formation and bone biomechanics. *Calcif Tissue Int.* 1997;61:S12–S14.

20. Agnusdei D, Camporeale F, Zacchei F, et al. Effects of ipriflavone on bone mass and bone remodeling in patients with established postmenopausal osteoporosis. *Curr Ther Res.* 1992;51:82–91.

21. Valente M, Bufalino L, Castiglione GN, et al. Effects of 1-year treatment with ipriflavone on bone in postmenopausal women with low bone mass. *Calcif Tissue Int.* 1994;54:377–380.

22. Agnusdei D, Crepaldi G, Isaia G, et al. A double-blind placebo-controlled trial of ipriflavone for prevention of postmenopausal spinal bone loss. *Calcif Tissue Int.* 1997;61:142–147.

23. Gennari C, Adami S, Agnusdei D, et al. Effect of chronic treatment with ipriflavone in postmenopausal women with low bone mass. *Calcif Tissue Int.* 1997;61:S19–S22.

24. Gennari C, Agnusdei D, Crepaldi G, et al. Effect of ipriflavone—a synthetic derivative of natural isoflavones—on bone mass loss in the early years after menopause. *Menopause.* 1998;5:9–15.

25. Kovacs AB. Efficacy of ipriflavone in the prevention and treatment of postmenopausal osteoporosis. *Agents Actions.* 1994;41:86–87.

26. Gambacciani M, Cappagli B, Piaggesi L, et al. Ipriflavone prevents the loss of bone mass in pharmacological menopause induced by GnRH-agonists. *Calcif Tissue Int.* 1997;61:S15–S18.

27. Hosking DJ, McClung MR, Ravin P, et al. Alendronate in the prevention of osteoporosis: EPIC study two-year results. *J Bone Miner Res.* 1996;11:S133.

28. Devogelaer JP, Broll H, Correa-Rotter R, et al. Oral alendronate induces progressive increases in bone mass of the spine, hip, and total body over 3 years in postmenopausal women with osteoporosis. *Bone.* 1996;18:141–150.

29. Avioli LV. The future of ipriflavone in the management of osteoporotic syndromes. *Calcif Tissue Int.* 1997;61:S33–S35.

30. Passeri M, Biondi M, Costi D, et al. Effects of 2-year therapy with ipriflavone in elderly women with established osteoporosis. *Ital J Miner Electrolyte Metab.* 1995;9:137–144.

31. Maugeri D, Panebianco J, Russo MS, et al. Ipriflavone treatment of senile osteoporosis: results of a multicenter, double-blind clinical trial of 2 years. *Arch Gerontol Geriatr.* 1994;19:252–263.

32. Agnusdei D, Zacchei F, Bigazzi S, et al. Metabolic and clinical effects of ipriflavone in established postmenopausal osteoporosis. *Drugs Expl Clin Res.* 1989;15:97–104.

33. Agnusdei D, Camporeale A, Zacchei F, et al. Effects of ipriflavone on bone mass and bone remodeling in patients with established postmenopausal osteoporosis. *Curr Ther Res.* 1992;51:82–91.

34. Scali G, Mansanti P, Zurlo A, et al. Analgesic effect of ipriflavone versus calcitonin in the treatment of osteoporotic vertebral pain. *Curr Ther Res.* 1991;49:1004–1010.

35. Moscarini M, Patacchiola F, Spacca G, et al. New perspectives in the treatment of postmenopausal osteoporosis: ipriflavone. *Gynecol Endocrinol.* 1994;8:203–207.

36. Melis GB, Paoletti AM, Bartolini R, et al. Ipriflavone and low doses of estrogens in the prevention of bone mineral loss in climacterium. *Bone Miner.* 1992;19(suppl):S49–S56.

37. Nozaki M, Hashimoto K, Inoue Y, et al. Treatment of bone loss in oophorectomized women with a combination of ipriflavone

and conjugated equine estrogen. *Int J Gynecol Obstet.* 1998;62:69–75.

38. Yamazaki I. Effect of ipriflavone on the response of uterus and thyroid to estrogen. *Life Sci.* 1986;38:757–764.

39. Agnusdei D, Bufalino L. Efficacy of ipriflavone in established osteoporosis and long-term safety. *Calcif Tissue Int.* 1997;61:S23–S27.

40. Melis G, Paoletti A, Cagnacci A, et al. Lack of any estrogenic effect of ipriflavone in postmenopausal women. *J Endocrinol Invest.* 1992;15:755–761.

41. Caltagirone S, Ranelletti RO, Rinelli A, et al. Interaction with type II estrogen binding sites and antiproliferative activity of tamoxifen and quercetin in human non-small-cell lung cancer. *Am J Respir Cell Mol Biol.* 1997;17: 51–59.

42. Ferrandina G, Almadori G, Maggiano N, et al. Growth-inhibitory effect of tamoxifen and quercetin and presence of type II estrogen binding sites in human laryngeal cancer cell lines and primary laryngeal tumors. *Int J Cancer.* 1998;77:747–754.

43. Kuiper GG, Lemmen JG, CarlssonB, et al. Interaction of estrogenic chemicals and phytoestrogens with estrogen receptor beta. *Endocrinology.* 1998;139:4252–4263.

44. Petilli M, Fiorelli G, Benvenuti S, et al. Interactions between ipriflavone and the estrogen receptor. *Calcif Tissue Int.* 1995;56:160–165.

Chapter 6
Other Important Nutrients for Your Bones

1. Feskanich D, Weber P, Willett WC, et al. Vitamin K intake and hip fractures in women: a prospective study. *Am J Clin Nutr.* 1999;69:74–79.

2. Weber P. The role of vitamins in the prevention of osteoporosis—a brief status report. *Int J Vitam Nutr Res.* 1999;69:194–7.

3. Hart JP, Catterall A, Dodds RA, et al. Circulating vitamin K_1 levels in fractured neck of femur. *Lancet.* 1984;2:283.

4. Hart JP, Shearer MJ, Klenerman L, et al. Electrochemical detection of depressed circulating levels of vitamin K_1 in osteoporosis. *J Clin Endocrinol Metab.* 1985;60:1268–1269.

5. Kanai T, Takagi T, Masuhiro K, et al. Serum vitamin K level and bone mineral density in postmenopausal women. *Int J Gynecol Obstet.* 1997;56:25–30.

6. Bitensky L, Hart JP, Catterall A, et al. Circulation vitamin K levels in patients with fractures. *J Bone Joint Surg Br.* 1988;70:663–664.

7. Hodges SJ, Pilkington MJ, Stamp TCB, et al. Depressed levels of circulating menaquinones in patients with osteoporotic fractures of the spine and femoral neck. *Bone.* 1991;12:387–389.

8. Booth SL, Tucker KL, Chen H, et al. Dietary vitamin K intakes are associated with hip fracture but not with bone mineral density in elderly men and women. *Am J Clin Nutr.* 2000;71:1201–1208.

9. Teomita A. Postmenopausal osteoporosis Ca kinetic study with vitamin K_2. *Clin Endocrinol (Japan).* 1971;19:731–736. Taken from: *N Engl J Med.* 1980;302:1460–1466.

10. Knapen MH, Jie KS, Hamulyak K, et al. Vitamin K-induced changes in markers for osteoblast activity and urinary calcium loss. *Calcif Tissue Int.* 1993;53:81–85.

11. Jie KS, Gijsbers BL, Knapen MH, et al. Effects of vitamin K and oral anticoagulants on urinary calcium excretion. *Br J Haematol.* 1993;83:100–104.

12. Knapen MH, Hamulyak K, Vermeer C. The effect of vitamin K supplementation on circulating osteocalcin (bone GLA protein) and urinary calcium excretion. *Ann Intern Med.* 1989;111:1001–1005.

13. Nurses' Health Study. *Am J Clin Nutr.* 1999;69:74–79.

14. Wallach S. Effects of magnesium on skeletal metabolism. *Magnes Trace Elem.* 1990;9:1–14.

15. Rude RK, Adams JS, Ryzen E, et al. Low serum concentrations of 1,25-dihydroxyvitamin D in human magnesium deficiency. *J Clin Endocrinol Metab.* 1985;61:933–940.

16. Hahn TJ. Parathyroid hormone, Calcitonin, Vitamin D, mineral and bone: Metabolism and Disorders. *Textbook of Endocrinology.* 3rd ed.; 1986:467.

17. Fatemi S, Ryzen E, Flores J, et al. Effect of experimental human magnesium depletion on parathyroid hormone secre-

tion and 1,25-dihydroxyvitamin D metabolism. *J Clin Endocrinol Metab.* 1991;73:1067–1072.

18. Iseri LT, French JH. Magnesium: nature's physiologic calcium blocker. *Am Heart J.* 1984;108:188–193.

19. Pao EM, Mickle S. Problem nutrients in the United States. *Food Technol.* 1981;35:58–69.

20. Bunker VW. The role of nutrition in osteoporosis. *Br J Biomed Sci.* 1994;51:228–240.

21. Marier JR. Magnesium content of the food supply in the modern-day world. *Magnesium.* 1986;5:1–8.

22. Durlach J, Bac Pierre, Durlach V, et al. Magnesium status and ageing: an update. *Magnes Res.* 1997;11:25–42.

23. Mountokalakis TD. Effects of aging, chronic disease, and multiple supplements on magnesium requirements. *Magnesium.* 1987;6:5–11.

24. Marier JR. Magnesium content of the food supply in the modern-day world. *Magnesium.* 1986;5:1–8.

25. Cohen L, Kitzes R. Infrared spectroscopy and magnesium content of bone mineral in osteoporotic women. *Isr J Med Sci.* 1981;17:1123–1125.

26. Angus RM, Sambrook PN, Pocock NA, et al. Dietary intake and bone mineral density. *Bone Miner.* 1988;4:265–275.

27. Tranquilli AL, Lucino E, Garzetti GG, et al. Calcium, phosphorus and magnesium intakes correlate with bone mineral content in postmenopausal women. *Gynecol Endocrinol.* 1994;8:55–58.

28. Ubbink JB, Vermaak WJ, Delport R, et al. Bio-availability of calcium and magnesium from magnesium citrate calcium malate. *S Afr Med J.* 1997;87:1271–1276.

29. Wallach S. Effects of magnesium on skeletal metabolism. *Magnem Trace Elem.* 1990;9:1–14.

30. Gaby A. *Preventing and Reversing Osteoporosis: Every Woman's Essential Guide.* Rocklin, CA: Prima Publishing; 1995:69.

31. Frank O, Jaslow SP, Thind I, et al. Superiority of periodic intramuscular vitamins over daily oral vitamins in maintaining nor-

mal vitamin titers in a geriatric population. *Am J Clin Nutr.* 1977;30:630.

32. Dodds RA, Catterall A, Bitensky L, et.al. Abnormalities in fracture healing induced by vitamin B_6-deficiency in rats. *Bone.* 1986;7:489–495.

33. Benke PH, Fleshood HL, Pitot HC. Osteoporotic bone disease in the pyridoxine-deficient rat. *Biochem Med.* 1972;6:526–535.

34. Kass-Annese B. Alternative therapies for menopause. *Clin Obstet Gynecol.* 2000;43:162–183

35. Brattstrom LE, Hultberg BL, Hardebo JE. Folic acid responsive postmenopausal homocysteinemia. *Metabolism.* 1985;34:1073–1077.

36. Moghadasian MH, McManus BM, Frohlich JJ. Homocysteine and coronary artery disease. *Arch Intern Med.* 1997;157:2299–2308.

37. Murray MT. *Encyclopedia of Nutritional Supplements: Essential Guide for Improving Health.* Rocklin, CA: Prima Publishing; 1996:109.

38. Parry G, Bredesen DE. Sensory neuropathy with low-dose pyridoxine. *Neurology.* 1985;35:1466–1468.

39. Strause L, Saltman P, Smith K, et al. Spinal bone loss in postmenopausal women supplemented with calcium and trace minerals. *Hum Nutr Clin Nutr.* 1994;124:1060–1064.

40. Werbach M. *Nutritional Influences on Illness.* New Caanan: Keats Publishing, Inc; 1987:466.

41. Amdur MO, Norris LC, Heuser GF. The need for manganese in bone development by the rat. *Proc Soc Exp Biol Med.* 1945;59:254–255.

42. Saltman PD, Strause LG. The role of trace minerals in osteoporosis. *J Am Coll Nutr.* 1993;12:384–389.

43. Nielson FH, Mullen LM, Gallagher SK. Effect of boron depletion and repletion on blood indicators of calcium status in humans fed a magnesium-low diet. *J Trace Elem Exp Med.* 1990;3:45–54.

44. Nielsen FH, Hunt CD, Mullen LM, et al. Effect of dietary boron on mineral, estrogen, and testosterone metabolism in postmenopausal women. *FASEB J.* 1987;1:394–397.

45. Beattie JH, Peace HS. The influence of a low-boron diet and boron supplementation on bone, major mineral and sex steroid metabolism in postmenopausal women. *Br J Nutr.* 1993;69:871–884.

46. Atik OS. Zinc and senile osteoporosis. *J Am Geriatr Soc.* 1983;31:790–791.

47. Werbach M. *Nutritional Influences on Illness.* New Caanan: Keats Publishing Inc; 1987:457–458.

48. Hoffman HN II, Phyliky RL, Fleming CR. Zinc-induced copper deficiency. *Gastroenterology.* 1988;94:508–512.

49. Sandstead HH. Requirements and toxicity of essential trace elements, illustrated by zinc and copper. *Am J Clin Nutr.* 1995;61(suppl):621S–624S.

50. Fosmire GJ. Zinc toxicity. *Am J Clin Nutr.* 1990;51:225–227.

51. Lim D, McKay M. Food-drug interactions. Drug Information Bulletin (UCLA Dept. of Pharmaceutical Services) 15(2):1995.

52. Drug evaluations subscription, vol.2 (section 13, chapter 5. Chicago: American Medical Association): Winter 1993.

53. Holt GA. *Food and Drug Interactions: A Professional's Guide to Protect You & Your Family.* Chicago: Precept Press; 1998:275, 284.

54. Reyes AJ, Olhaberry JV, Leary WP, et al. Urinary zinc excretion, diuretics, zinc deficiency and some side effects of diuretics. *S Afr Med J.* 1983;64:936–941.

55. Evans-Eaton J, McIlrath EM, Jackson WE, et al. Copper supplementation and the maintenance of bone mineral density in middle-aged women. *J Trace Elem Exp Med.* 1996;9:87.

56. Wilson T, Katz JM, Gray DH. Inhibition of active bone resorption by copper. *Calcif Tissue Int.* 1981;33:35–39.

57. Werbach M. *Foundations of Nutritional Medicine: A Sourcebook of Clinical Research.* Tarzana, CA: Third Line Press; 1997:169–171, 206.

58. [No author listed]. Silicon and bone formation. *Nutr Rev.* 1980;38:194–195.

Chapter 7
Exercise, Diet, and Lifestyle:
What You Can Do to Protect Your Bones

1. Ernst E. Can exercise prevent postmenopausal osteoporosis? *Br J Sports Med.* 1994;28:5–6.

2. Dalen N, Olsson KE. Bone mineral content and physical activity. *Acta Orthop Scand.* 1974;45:170–174.

3. Law MR, Wald NJ, Meade TW. Strategies for prevention of osteoporosis and hip fracture. *Br Med J.* 1991;303:453–459.

4. Bravo G, Gauthier P, Roy PM, et al. Impact of a 12-month exercise program on the physical and psychological health of osteopenic women. *JAGS.* 1996;44:756–762.

5. Ayalon J, Simkin A, Leichter I, et al. Dynamic bone loading exercises for postmenopausal women: Effect on the density of the distal radius. *Arch Phys Med Rehabil.* 1987;68:280–283.

6. Krolner B, Toft B, Nielsen SP, et al. Physical exercise as prophylaxis against involutional vertebral bone loss: a controlled study. *Clin Sci.* 1983;64:541–546.

7. Debenedette V. Swimming may increase bone density. *Phys Sports Med.* 1987;10:72–82.

8. Hoshi A, Watanabe H, Chiba M, et al. Bone density and mechanical properties in femoral bone of swim loaded aged mice. *Biomed Environ Sci.* 1998;11:243–250.

9. Taaffe DR, Marcus R. Regional and total body bone mineral density in elite collegiate male swimmers. *J Sports Med Phys Fitness.* 1999;39:154–159.

10. Radetti G, Frizzera S, Castellan C, et al. Bone density in swimmers [in Italian]. *Pediatr Med Chir.* 1992;14:521–522.

11. Layne JE, Nelson ME. The effects of progressive resistance training on bone density: a review. *Med Sci Sports Exerc.* 1999;31:25–30.

12. Shank FR, Park YK, Harland BF, et al. Perspectives of the Food and Drug Administration on dietary sodium. *J Am Diet Assoc.* 1982;80:29–35.

13. American Dietetic Association. The Sodium Story. 1991.

14. Goulding A, Lim PE. Effects of varying dietary salt intake on the fasting urinary excretion of sodium, calcium, and hydroxyproline in young women. *N Engl J Med.* 1983;96:853–862.

15. Devine A, Criddle RA, Dick IM, et al. A longitudinal study of the effect of sodium and calcium intakes on regional bone density in postmenopausal women. *Am J Clin Nutr.* 1995;62:740–745.

16. Wyshak G, Frisch R. Carbonated beverages, dietary calcium, the dietary calcium/phosphorus ratio, and bone fractures in girls and boys. *J Adolesc Health.* 1994;15:210–215.

17. Portale A, Halloran B, Morris R. Physiologic regulation of the serum concentration of 1,25-dihydroxyvitamin D by phosphorus in normal men. *J Clin Invest.* 1989;83:1494–1499.

18. Mets JA, Anderson JJ. Intakes of calcium, phosphorus, and protein, and physical activity level are related to radial bone mass in young adult women. *Am J Clin Nutr.* 1993;56:537–542.

19. Calvo M, Kumar R. Persistently elevated parathyroid hormone secretion and action in young women after four weeks of ingesting high phosphorus, low calcium diets. *J Clin Endocrinol Metab.* 1990;70:1334–1339.

20. Calvo M, Kumar H. Elevated secretion and action of serum parathyroid hormone in young adults consuming high phosphorus, low calcium diets assembled from common foods. *J Clin Endocrinol Met.* 1988;66:823–830.

21. Calvo M. Dietary phosphorus, calcium metabolism and bone. *J Nutr.* 1993;123:1627–1633.

22. Silverberg S, Shane E, De La Cruz L, et al. Abnormalities in parathyroid hormone secretion and 1,25-dihydroxyvitamin D_3 formation in women with osteoprosis. *N Engl J Med.* 1989;320:277–281.

23. Pennington J, Church H. *Food Values of Portions Commonly Used.* New York: Harper & Row; 1985.

Chapter 8
Progesterone: An Option for Osteoporosis?

1. Mack TH, Pike MC, Henderson BE, et al. Estrogens and endometrial cancer in a retirement community. *N Engl J Med.* 1976;294:1262–1267.

2. Smith DC, Prentice R, Thompson DJ, et al. Association of exogenous estrogen and endometrial carcinoma. *N Engl J Med.* 1975;293:1164–1167.

3. Gambrel D. Clinical use of progestins in the menopausal patient. *J Reprod Med.* 1982;27:8.

4. Gambrell RD. The role of hormones in endometrial cancer. *South Med J.* 1978;71:1280.

5. Fahraeus L. The effects of estradiol on blood lipids and lipoproteins in post-menopausal women. *Obstet Gynecol.* 1988;72:188.

6. Gambrell RD. Role of hormones in the etiology and prevention of endometrial breast cancer. *Acta Obstet Gynecol Scand.* 1982;106;37.

7. Ross RK, Pike MC. Effect of hormone replacement therapy on breast cancer risk: estrogen versus estrogen plus progestin. *J Natl Cancer Inst.* 2000;92:1100A–11101.

8. Schairer C, Lubin J Troisi R, et al. Menopausal estrogen and estrogen-progestin replacement therapy and breast cancer risk. *JAMA.* 2000;283:485–491.

9. Martorano J. Differentiating between natural progesterone and synthetic progestogens: clinical implications for premenstrual syndrome management. *Compr Ther.* 1993;19:96–98.

10. McAuley JW, Kroboth FJ, Kroboth PD. Oral administration of micronized progesterone: a review and more experience. *Pharmacotherapy.* 1996;16:453–457.

11. Hargrove JT, Maxson WS, Wentz AC, et al. Menopausal hormone replacement therapy with continuous oral micronized estradiol and progesterone. *Obstet Gynecol.* 1989;73:606–612.

12. Dennerstein L, Spencer-Gardner C, Gotts G, et al. Progesterone and the premenstrual syndrome: a double-blind crossover trial. *Br Med J.* 1985;290:1617–1621.

13. Erny R, Pigne A, Prouvost C, et al. The effects of oral administration of progesterone for premature labor. *Am J Obstet Gynecol.* 1986;154:525–529.

14. Devroey P, Palermo G, Bourgain C, et al. Progesterone administration in patients with absent ovaries. *Int J Fertil.* 1989;34:188–193.

15. Freeman EW, Rickels K, Sondheimer SJ, et al. A double-blind trial of oral progesterone, alprazolam, and placebo in treatment of severe premenstrual syndrome. *JAMA.* 1995;274:51–57.

16. McNeeley SG Jr, Schinfeld JS, Stovall TG, et al. Prevention of osteoporosis by medroxyprogesterone acetate in post-menopausal women. *Int J Gynaecol Obstet.* 1991;34:253–256.

17. Lindsay R, Hart DM, Purdie D, et al. Comparative effects of oestrogen and a progestogen on bone loss in postmenopausal women. *Clin Sci Mol Med.* 1978;54:193.

18. McNeeley SG Jr, Schinfeld JS, Stovall TG, et al. Prevention of osteoporosis by medroxyprogesterone acetate in postmenopausal women. *Int J Gynaecol Obstet.* 1991;34:253–256.

19. Leonetti HB, Longo S, Anasti JN. Transdermal progesterone cream for vasomotor symptoms and postmenopausal bone loss. *Obstet Gynecol.* 1999;94:225–228.

20. Colditz GA, Hankinson SE, Hunter DJ, et al. The use of estrogens and progestins and the risk of breast cancer and post-menopausal women. *N Engl J Med.* 1995;332:1589–1593.

21. Fugh-Berman A. Progesterone cream for osteoporosis. *Alt Ther Women's Health.* 1999;1:33–40.

22. Martorano J. Differentiating between natural progesterone and synthetic progestogens: clinical implications for premenstrual syndrome management. *Compr Ther.* 1993;19:96–98.

23. Hargrove JT, Maxson WS, Wentz AC, et al. Menopausal hormone replacement therapy with continuous oral micronized estradiol and progesterone. *Obstet Gynecol.* 1989;73:606.

24. Gillet JY, Andre G, Faguer B, et al. Induction of amenorrhea during hormone replacement therapy: optimal micronized progesterone dose: a multicenter study. *Maturitas.* 1994;19:103.

Chapter 9
Conventional Treatments for Osteoporosis

1. Genant HK, Baylink DJ, Gallagher JC. Estrogens in the prevention of osteoporosis in postmenopausal women. *Am J Obstet Gynecol.* 1989;161:1842–1846.

2. Delmas PD. Hormone replacement therapy in the prevention and treatment of osteoporosis. *Osteoporos Int.* 1997;7(suppl 1):S3–S7.

3. Hulley S, Grady D, Bush T, et al. Randomized trial of estrogen plus progestin for secondary prevention of coronary heart disease in postmenopausal women. *JAMA.* 1998;280:605–613.

4. Colditz GA, Hankinson SE, Hunter DJ, et al. The use of estrogens and progestins and the risk of breast cancer in postmenopausal women. *N Engl J Med.* 1995;332:1589–1593.

5. Gapstur SM, Morrow M, Sellers TA. Hormone replacement therapy and risk of breast cancer with a favorable histology: results of the Iowa Women's Health Study. *JAMA.* 1999;281:2091–2097.

6. Paganini-Hill A. Morbidity and mortality changes with estrogen replacement therapy. In: Lobo R, ed. Treatment of the postmenopausal woman, basic and clinical aspects. New York: Raven Press. 1994;399.

7. Colditz GA, Hankinson SE, Hunter DJ, et al. The use of estrogens and progestins and the risk of breast cancer in postmenopausal women. *N Engl J Med.* 1995;332:1589–1593.

8. Hulley S, Grady D, Bush T, et al. Randomized trial of estrogen plus progestin for secondary prevention of coronary heart disease in postmenopausal women. *JAMA.* 1998;280:605–613.

9. Paganini-Hill A. Morbidity and mortality changes with estrogen replacement therapy. In: Lobo R, ed. Treatment of the postmenopausal woman, basic and clinical aspects. New York: Raven Press. 1994;399.

10. Petitti DB, Sidney S, Perlman JA. Increased risk of cholecystectomy in users of supplemental estrogen. *Gastroenterology.* 1988;94:91–95.

11. Cummings SR, Eckert S, Krueger KA, et al. The effect of raloxifene on risk of breast cancer in postmenopausal women: results from the MORE randomized trial. Multiple Outcomes of Raloxifene Evaluation. *JAMA.* 1999;281:2189–2197.

12. Ettinger B, Black DM, Mitlak BH, et al. Reduction of vertebral fracture risk in postmenopausal women with osteoporosis treated with raloxifene: results from a 3-year randomized clini-

cal trial. Multiple Outcomes of Raloxifene Evaluation (MORE) Investigators. *JAMA.* 1999;282:637–645.

13. Liberman UA, Weiss SR, Broll J, et al. Effect of oral alendronate on bone mineral density and the incidence of fractures in postmenopausal osteoporosis. *N Engl J Med.* 1995;333:1437–1443.

14. Tucci J, Tonino R, Emkey RD. Effect of three years of oral alendronate treatment in postmenopausal women with osteoporosis. *Am J Med.* 1996;101:488–501.

15. Bellantoni M. Osteoporosis prevention and treatment. *Am Fam Physician.* 1996;54:986–992.

16. Love R, Mazess RB, Barden HS, et al. Effects of tamoxifen on bone mineral density in postmenopausal women with breast cancer. *N Engl J Med.* 1992;326:852–856.

17. Kleerekoper M. The role of fluoride in the prevention of osteoporosis. *Endocrinol Metab Clin North Am.* 1998;27:441–451.

Chapter 10
Evaluation and Screening for Osteoporosis

1. Schreiber L, Torregrosa T. Evaluation and treatment of postmenopausal osteoporosis. *Semin Arthritis Rheum.* 1998;2:245–261.

Index

Abdominal pain from alendronate, 139

ACE inhibitors and zinc deficiency, 100

Acne
from estrogen, 130
from progestins, 126

Adolescents. *See* Children

Aerobic exercise. *See* Exercise

African-Americans and osteoporosis risk, 20–21

Age
bone loss and, 7–9
early menopause and osteoporosis risk, 19–20, 23, 34–35
late menarche and osteoporosis risk, 18, 19–20, 34–35
life cycle of bones, 6–8
magnesium deficiency and, 91
osteoporosis prevalence and, xi, 2
osteoporosis risk and, 1, 17, 18
vitamin D production and, 52

Alcohol
magnesium deficiency and, 91, 92
osteoporosis risk and, 19, 23, 27–28, 103

Alendronate (Fosamax)
benefits of, 14, 139
ipriflavone compared to, 79–80
safety issues, 139
side effects, 139
table summarizing benefits and risks, 130

Alkaline phosphotase, 90

Aluminum-containing antacids. *See* Antacids

Alzheimer's disease and ERT, 133

Amen (medroxyprogesterone acetate), 119. *See also* Progestins

Amenorrhea from strenuous exercise, 35–36, 108–109

American Journal of Public Health, 50

American Society for Bone and Mineral Research, 60

Amiloride, zinc safety issues, 100

Ancestry and osteoporosis risk, 18, 20–21

Anemia
sodium fluoride safety issues, 131, 142
zinc safety issues, 100

Anorexia nervosa and osteoporosis risk, 23, 36

Antacids
calcium safety issues, 66
copper deficiency and, 101
manganese absorption and, 98
osteoporosis risk and, 27

Antibiotics
calcium interference with, 65
zinc interference with, 100

Anticoagulants
calcium and vitamin supplementation with, 67
vitamin K safety issues, 90

Anticonvulsant medications
calcium absorption and, 63–64
calcium and vitamin D with, 56

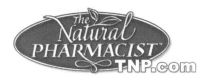

About the Authors

Sheila Dunn-Merritt, N.D., has been in private practice since 1983. One of the first graduates of Bastyr University, she has been a pioneer in the field of natural medicine. In addition to her private practice in Bellevue, Washington, Dr. Dunn-Merritt lectures extensively to consumers in the Seattle area on health care topics such as menopause, optimal aging, dealing with depression naturally, and detoxification for health.

Lyn Patrick, N.D., has been in private practice as both an acupuncturist and licensed naturopathic physician for 15 years. She is an author and associate editor for the MEDLINE-indexed, peer-reviewed journal, *Alternative Medicine Review*. Dr. Patrick has published articles and spoken nationally on the subject of nicotine addiction treatment, osteoporosis, and complementary and alternative treatment for HIV/AIDS and Hepatitis C.

About the Editors

Carol Poole is an editor and author of natural health-related material for TNP.com. She is also editor of the Osteoporosis Community information at TNP.com.

Andrea M. Girman, M.D., M.P.H., is Associate Medical Director of TNP.com. A graduate of the Johns Hopkins University School of Medicine and Pediatric residency program, she also holds a Masters of Public Health degree from the JHU School of Hygiene and Public Health. An avid proponent of women's health issues, education, and prevention, Dr. Girman's primary focus since clinical training has been on scientific accuracy in both traditional and natural health information.

About the Series Editors

Steven Bratman, M.D., is Medical Director of TNP.com. Dr. Bratman is both a strong proponent and vocal critic of alternative treatment, and he believes that alternative medicine has both strengths and weaknesses, just like conventional medicine. This even-handed critique has made him a trusted party on both sides of the debate.

Dr. Bratman has studied acupuncture, herbology, nutrition, massage, osteopathic manipulation, and body-oriented psychotherapy, and he has worked closely with a wide variety of alternative practitioners.

He has been an expert consultant to the State of Washington Medical Board, the Colorado Board of Medical Examiners, and the Texas State Board of Medical Examiners, evaluating disciplinary cases involving alternative medicine.

He has published articles in numerous national magazines, including *Yoga Journal, Utne Reader, Bottom-line Health, Delicious,* and the peer-reviewed *Alternative Therapies in Health and Medicine.* He has been a contributor to America Online's Alternative Medicine forum and he authored a monthly column in *Your Health.*

His books include *The Alternative Medicine Sourcebook: A Realistic Evaluation of Alternative Healing Methods* (1997), *The Alternative Medicine Ratings Guide: An Expert Panel Ranks the Best Alternative Treatments for Over 80 Conditions* (Prima Health, 1998), the professional text *Clinical Evaluation of Medicinal Herbs and Other Therapeutic Natural Products* (Prima Health, 1999), and the following titles in *The Natural Pharmacist* series: *Your Complete Guide to Herbs* (Prima Health, 1999), *Your Complete Guide to Illnesses and their Natural Remedies* (Prima Health, 1999), *Natural Health Bible* (Prima Health, 1999), and *St. John's Wort and Depression* (Prima Health, 1999).

David J. Kroll, Ph.D., is a professor of pharmacology and toxicology at the University of Colorado School of Pharmacy and a consultant for pharmacists, physicians, and alternative practitioners on the indications and cautions for herbal medicine use. He received a degree in toxicology from the Philadelphia College of Pharmacy and Science and obtained his Ph.D. from the University of Florida College of Medicine.

Dr. Kroll has lectured widely and has published articles in a number of medical journals, abstracts, and newsletters. He is also co-author of both *Natural Health Bible* and the professional text *Clinical Evaluation of Medicinal Herbs and Other Therapeutic Natural Products.*